Understanding Health Services

Understanding Public Health Series

Series editors: Nicki Thorogood and Rosalind Plowman, London School of Hygiene & Tropical Medicine (previous edition edited by Nick Black and Rosalind Raine).

Throughout the world, recognition of the importance of public health to sustainable, safe, and healthy societies is growing. The achievements of public health in nineteenth-century Europe were for much of the twentieth century overshadowed by advances in personal care, in particular in hospital care. Now, with the dawning of a new century, there is increasing understanding of the inevitable limits of individual health care and of the need to complement such services with effective public health strategies. Major improvements in people's health will come from controlling communicable diseases, eradicating environmental hazards, improving people's diets, and enhancing the availability and quality of effective health care. To achieve this, every country needs a cadre of knowledgeable public health practitioners with social, political, and organizational skills to lead and bring about changes at international, national, and local levels.

This is one of a series of books that provides a foundation for those wishing to join in and contribute to the twenty-first-century regeneration of public health, helping to put the concerns and perspectives of public health at the heart of policy-making and service provision. While each book stands alone, together they provide a comprehensive account of the three main aims of public health: protecting the public from environmental hazards, improving the health of the public, and ensuring high-quality health services are available to all. Some of the books focus on methods, others on key topics. They have been written by staff at the London School of Hygiene & Tropical Medicine with considerable experience of teaching public health to students from low-, middle-, and high-income countries. Much of the material has been developed and tested with postgraduate students both in face-to-face teaching and through distance learning.

The books are designed for self-directed learning. Each chapter has explicit learning objectives, key terms are highlighted, and the text contains many activities to enable the reader to test their own understanding of the ideas and material covered. Written in a clear and accessible style, the series will be essential reading for students taking postgraduate courses in public health and will also be of interest to public health practitioners and policy-makers.

Titles in the series

Analytical models for decision making: Colin Sanderson and Reinhold Gruen
Conflict and health: Natasha Howard, Egbert Sondorp, and Annemarie Ter Veen (eds.)
Controlling communicable disease: Norman Noah
Economic analysis for management and policy: Stephen Jan, Lilani Kumaranayake, Jenny Roberts, Kara Hanson, and Kate Archibald
Economic evaluation: Julia Fox-Rushby and John Cairns (eds.)
Environmental epidemiology: Paul Wilkinson (ed.)
Environmental health policy: Megan Landon and Tony Fletcher
Environment, health and sustainable development, second edition: Emma Hutchinson and Sari Kovats
Financial management in health services: Reinhold Gruen and Anne Howarth
Health care evaluation, second edition: Carmen Tsang and David Cromwell (eds.)
Health promotion practice, second edition: Will Nutland and Liza Cragg (eds.)
Health promotion theory, second edition: Liza Cragg, Maggie Davies, and Wendy MacDowall (eds.)
Introduction to epidemiology, second edition: Ilona Carneiro and Natasha Howard
Introduction to health economics, second edition: Lorna Guinness and Virginia Wiseman (eds.)
Issues in public health, second edition: Fiona Sim and Martin McKee (eds.)
Making health policy, second edition: Kent Buse, Nicholas Mays, and Gill Walt
Managing health services: Nick Goodwin, Reinhold Gruen, and Valerie Iles
Medical anthropology: Robert Pool and Wenzel Geissler
Principles of social research, second edition: Mary Alison Durand and Tracey Chantler (eds.)
Public health in history: Virginia Berridge, Martin Gorsky, and Alex Mold
Sexual health: A public health perspective: Kay Wellings, Kirstin Mitchell, and Martine Collumbien (eds.)

Forthcoming titles

Applied communicable disease control: Liza Cragg, Will Nutland and R. Gregory Thomas-Reilly

Understanding Health Services

Second edition

İpek Gürol-Urgancı, Fiona Campbell
and Nick Black

 Open University Press

Open University Press
McGraw-Hill Education
8th Floor
338 Euston Road
London
NW1 3BH

email: enquiries@openup.co.uk
world wide web: www.mheducation.co.uk

and Two Penn Plaza, New York, NY 10121-2289, USA

First published 2005
First published in this second edition 2017

A catalogue record of this book is available from the British Library

ISBN-13: 978-0-33-526214-4
ISBN-10: 0-33-526214-7
eISBN: 978-0-33-526215-1

Library of Congress Cataloging-in-Publication Data
CIP data applied for

Typeset by Transforma Pvt. Ltd., Chennai, India

Printed and bound by CPI Group (UK) Ltd, Croydon, CR0 4YY

Praise page

"This excellent book provides an ideal background to understanding how health services work and how they can be studied. Not tied to any particular country, it includes key chapters on how health services have developed and are organised, need and demand, the role of health professionals, and measuring and improving quality of care. The book is ideal reading for students on Masters courses in public health and related subjects from high-, middle- and low-income countries and includes learning objectives and exercises in each chapter which can be completed individually or used for discussion. Strongly recommended."

Martin Roland, Emeritus Professor of Health
Services Research, University of Cambridge, UK

"Health services are central to attaining high levels of population health and providing those services consumes a substantial share of our financial resources. This book provides a splendid introduction to many of the key building blocks including medical knowledge and other key inputs, payment and other factors that influence utilization, and in turn quality of care and outcomes. The learning objectives are a wonderful aid for self-directed learning as are the directed activities and feedback, the text is lucid and the main concepts are very easy to access. This is a great book for someone looking to develop a broad understanding of health services. I will be surprised if it does not become a classic. It will surely be at the top of my list of recommended readings for my own students."

Arnold M Epstein, John H Foster Professor and Chair,
Department of Health Policy and Management,
Harvard School of Public Health, USA

Contents

List of figures and tables   ix
Acknowledgements   xi
Overview of the book   xiii

Section 1: Introduction   **1**

1 A systems approach to health services   3
2 Formal and lay care   21

Section 2: Inputs to health care   **35**

3 Diseases and medical knowledge   37
4 Medical paradigms   52
5 Health care professionals   61
6 Funding health care   81

Section 3: Processes of health care   **105**

7 Need, demand, and use   107
8 Users of health care   133
9 Paying providers   158

Section 4: Outcomes and quality of health care   **175**

10 Quality of health services   177
11 Defining good quality health services   196
12 Quality assessment   208
13 Improving quality of care   226

Glossary   240
Index   246

List of figures and tables

Figures

2.1 Formal and lay care   23
5.1 Factors affecting migration   77
6.1 Universal coverage 'cube'   84
6.2 Expenditure on health by type of financing, 2013   86
6.3 Out-of-pocket expenditure on health as a percentage of total expenditure on health, 2013   87
6.4 Impoverishment and catastrophic health expenditure headcount by country income   89
7.1 A conceptual model of need, demand, and use   108
7.2 The clinical iceberg   111
7.3 Need, demand, and supply: influences and overlaps   114
7.4 Information sources and need, demand, and supply   115
7.5 Emergency admission rates for ambulatory care-sensitive conditions   120
7.6a Activity   121
7.6b Activity feedback   122
7.7 Variations in health care expenditures by age groups   124
7.8 Rates of common surgical procedures among Medicare patients for 306 referral regions   127
8.1 Ladder of participation   146
10.1 Aspects of health status using the example of benign prostatic hyperplasia   184
10.2 Quality management cycle   194
11.1 The environmental turbulence experienced by policy-makers   202
12.1 Hospital-wide standardized mortality ratios for 17 hospital trusts in the East of England   219
12.2 Funnel plot of standardized mortality ratios for adult critical care units in the UK in 2013   220
13.1 Impact of use of decision aids on demand for certain surgical operations in nine US studies and two UK studies   230

Tables

1.1 Examples from England of the nine historical factors that
shape health services   8
3.1 Pharmaceutical consumption in the UK and Germany:
defined daily doses in 1990   50
5.1 Key aspects of professional power   65
5.2 Arguments for and against professional autonomy   71
5.3 Professionalism, managerialism, and hybrid roles   75
5.4 Typology of professional elites   75
7.1 Categories of medical services   129
8.1 Relative importance of patient satisfaction factors and
frequency of negative responses   138
8.2 Parsons' doctor and patient privileges and obligations   141
8.3 Six collective health care decisions for which there is a
potential role for public input   149
9.1 Types of payment mechanisms   161
12.1 Top ten countries according to the WHO index measure
of health system quality   216

Acknowledgements

The authors would like to acknowledge the important contributions made by colleagues who developed the first edition of the book, the original lectures and teaching material at the London School of Hygiene and Tropical Medicine on which some of the contents are based: Reinhold Gruen (first edition author), Judith Green (Chapter 5), Josephine Borghi (Chapter 6), Alicia Renado (Chapter 8), and Mylene Lagarde (Chapter 9). The authors would also like to acknowledge the contribution of Lorelei Jones and the *Understanding Public Health* Series Editors, Rosalind Plowman and Nicki Thorogood, for reviewing the entire manuscript; and Josephine Borghi for reviewing Chapter 6.

Open University Press and the London School of Hygiene & Tropical Medicine have made every effort to obtain permission from copyright holders to reproduce material in this book and to acknowledge these sources correctly. Any omissions brought to our attention will be remedied in future editions.

Overview of the book

Introduction

Health services are an important aspect of public health and encompass the full range of activities with a primary intent to improve and maintain health. Your interest in health services may be as a clinician, a policy-maker or a manager. In this book, you will be introduced to the main concepts, historical factors, and contemporary discussions relating to the services to deliver quality health care, as a foundation for further study.

Why study health services?

There are a number of reasons why it is important to study health services. In the first instance, health is of primary importance to most people, and health services have an important role in contributing to maintaining and improving people's health. At the same time, there remains uncertainty as to the effectiveness, humanity, equity, and efficiency of many interventions, and there is a need to make health care professionals and services more accountable to the public. Expenditure on health care also represents a large and growing proportion of national budgets and health services are a major employer. Finally, the medical-industrial complex that supplies health services is a major power and influence on national governments and international organizations. You will look at these areas in more detail in the 'Introduction' section of the book.

The scope of this book

No single discipline can provide a full account of how and why health services are the way they are. This book provides you with a series of conceptual frameworks which help to explain the complexity. It demonstrates the need for a multidisciplinary approach to understanding health services and the contributions that medicine, sociology, economics, history, and epidemiology make. It also shows how it is necessary to consider health services on three levels: the micro level of the individual patient and their experiences; the meso level of how health care organizations such as health centres and hospitals work; and the macro level of regional and national institutions such as governments and health insurance bodies.

Many of the themes raised in this book are developed in companion volumes. The aim of this volume is to provide an overview that will help you place specific aspects of health services in a wider context.

You will have adopted your own view on health services, based on your professional background and experience. This view will help you as you work through the book. However, no specialist knowledge is required. The approach taken will broaden your view on health services and explain why health services are the way they are.

The concepts presented rarely take the form of exact definitions, such as you come across in statistics and epidemiology or when studying physical sciences. Rather, they should help you interpret complex issues and form your perspective on health services.

The structure of the book

This book follows the conceptual outline of the 'Health Services' Module taught at the London School of Hygiene & Tropical Medicine. It is based on the materials presented in the lectures and seminars of the face-to-face course, which have been adapted for distance learning.

The book is structured around a simple conceptual framework. It starts by looking at the inputs to health care, goes on to consider the processes of care, and then discusses the outcomes. Finally, you consider how the quality of health care can be assessed and improved.

The four sections, and the 13 chapters within them, are shown on the book's contents page. Each chapter includes:

- An overview
- A list of learning objectives
- A list of key terms
- A range of activities
- Feedback on activities
- A summary
- References.

Although examples and case studies in this book are balanced between low-, middle-, and high-income countries, you should be aware that much of the theory on health services has been developed in high-income countries.

The following description of the section and chapter contents will give you an idea of what you will be reading.

Section 1: Introduction

Chapter 1 will introduce you to health services. It explains the rationale for using a systems approach to the analysis of health services, and considers the principal challenges facing health services. Like most books in this area, you will be reading and learning principally about formal health care. However, there is also a critical role for informal or lay care, and you will consider the contribution of lay care and its relationship to formal care in Chapter 2.

Section 2: Inputs to health care

Chapters 3 and 4 provide a conceptual framework for understanding how medical knowledge shapes a key input to health care, that of patients and their diseases. In Chapter 5, you will consider a second input, that of staff. You will explore some of the contemporary challenges facing the health care professions. In Chapter 6, you will learn about the other essential input, finance.

Section 3: Processes of health care

In this section, you will focus first on the concepts of need, demand, and use. In Chapter 7, you will learn how to conceptualize the need for health care and examine which factors influence utilization of health services. Chapter 8 introduces you to the various roles played by users of health services, as patients, as consumers, and as members of the public participating in health care issues. In Chapter 9, you will learn about various payment mechanisms for individual practitioners and organizations.

Section 4: Outcomes and quality of health care

The fourth section focuses on managing the quality of health services. In Chapter 10, you will learn about outcomes, how to define and measure them, and the characteristics of a good measure. Chapters 11 to 13 consider how high quality can be defined, how the performance of health services can be assessed, and finally how practice and policy can be changed to improve quality.

A variety of activities are employed to help your understanding and learning of the topics and ideas covered. These include:

- Reflection on your own knowledge and experience.
- Questions based on reading key articles or relevant research papers.
- Analyses of quantitative or qualitative data.

SECTION 1

Introduction

A systems approach to health services

Overview

This chapter will introduce you to health services and why it is important to study them. You will look at the range of activities that make up health care and be introduced to a systems approach to looking at health services. You will explore how history has shaped health services before looking at some contemporary challenges facing a range of countries. Finally, you will look at the role of health services research in helping to understand how to improve health care.

Learning objectives

After working through this chapter, you will be able to:

- understand the range of activities included in health care
- understand what is meant by health services and why it is an important area of study
- understand a systems approach to health services
- understand how history has shaped health services
- analyse the factors influencing change and reform in health care
- understand contemporary challenges to health services
- outline the contribution of health services research to the organization and management of health services

Key terms

Corporate rationalizers: A contemporary approach to management in which the organization (corporation) attempts to dominate professional autonomy through the use of measurement and data.

Environmental turbulence: The ever-changing external pressures on an organization and its managers, such as legislation, the national economy, professional associations and trades unions, and public opinion.

Health services research (HSR): A multidisciplinary activity to improve the quality, organization, and management of health services. HSR is not itself a discipline.

Inputs: The resources needed by a system.

Outcomes: Change in status as a result of the system processes (in the health services context, the change in health status as a result of care).

Outputs: A combination of the processes and outcomes that constitute the total production of a system.

Payers: The people who provide funds to pay for health care.

Processes: The use of resources or the activity within a system.

Professional autonomy: The freedom that professionals have to make decisions without being 'accountable' to their employers or the state.

Prospective payment: Paying providers before any care is delivered, usually on the basis of capitation payments or contracts.

Providers: Organizations (hospitals, health centres) or individuals (community nurses) who provide formal or informal care.

Purchasers: Those who purchase health services from providers on behalf of those eligible to use health care.

Retrospective payment: Paying providers for any work they have undertaken, with no agreement in advance.

System: A model of a whole entity, reflecting the relationship between its elements at different levels of complexity.

What is meant by health services?

In thinking about health care, you may immediately consider it in quite narrow terms, such as curative services, and doctors and nurses, hospitals and clinics. However, health care encompasses a wide spectrum of activities covering health promotion, prevention of disease, rehabilitation and care, as well as cure. In some cases, it can also include custody.

Since the influences on health are so diverse, it can sometimes be difficult to draw the boundary around what we mean by health services. For the purposes of this book, health services are defined as encompassing *the full range of activities with a primary intent to improve and maintain health*. This definition, however, excludes a number of areas known to have a major impact on health, such as education, housing, and employment policies, which have goals in their own right beyond health. These factors are important social determinants of health, rather than aspects of health services.

In thinking about health services, it is important to consider where services are directed. Health services may be directed at the individual or they may be directed at the population. There is often a tension between these two aims. In many contexts there will also be two workforces to accommodate these two services and the necessary tension between them.

Health care is also provided at different *levels* – primary, secondary, and tertiary – and you will explore these levels of care in more detail in the next chapter.

Given the breadth of health care, large numbers of people are engaged in supporting health, beyond those working in hospitals and clinics. These workers may be formal or lay (informal) health care workers. You will also explore the distinction between formal and lay care in the next chapter.

Why study health services?

There are many reasons to study health services. In the first instance, health is of primary importance to most people. Although many factors contribute to the health of an individual, including lifestyle factors and social and environmental conditions (Dahlgren and Whitehead, 1991), health services have an important role in maintaining and improving people's health.

However, large disparities remain in population health between and within countries, and there is uncertainty regarding the effectiveness, humanity, equity, and efficiency of many interventions. Understanding how to improve health services is therefore critical. Often, it is factors within the service that are inhibiting improvement. For example, health professionals continue to dominate the decisions about health services, often limiting the options for change that might be considered. There is a need to improve accountability between health care professionals and the populations they serve.

There is also a need to consider the cost of health services. Expenditure on health care represents a large proportion of national budgets. In a number of high-income countries, the costs of health care may account for a significant percentage of gross domestic product (GDP). In the USA, 17 per cent of GDP is currently spent on health care, while in the UK this figure is nearer 9 per cent (WHO, 2015). In low-income countries, the percentage of GDP spent on health is often lower but can still present a challenge for policy makers. Expenditure on health care is also rising. The challenge for all countries, no matter what their income level, is to provide high quality health services within available resources.

Health services are also a major employer of staff in a country and have a role to play beyond the provision of health care. In addition, there are many industries and companies that are directly associated with health services. These include drug companies, private insurance firms, and others. All have a vested interest in how health services are organized. These interests may not always align with the interest of patients.

These factors make health care an important political issue. Health has been used as a key political election issue in many countries. For example, in Uganda, President Museveni's decision to remove user fees was a highly popular move in the 2001 election (Moat and Abelson, 2011). In the USA, the Affordable Care Act ('Obamacare') was a key political issue during President Obama's administration, while parties in the 2015 UK general election made the National Health Service (NHS) a chief commitment in their election pledges.

A systems approach to health services

In looking at health services, it helps to consider them from a systems perspective. A system has:

- a purpose or mission;
- decision-making processes that are themselves systems – these interact so that their effects can be transmitted throughout the system;
- resources that can be used by the decision-making process;
- some guarantee of continuity.

Also:

- its performance can be measured; and
- it exists in wider systems and/or environments with which it interacts but from which it is separated.

There are many different ways of describing a system, but whatever approach you choose, you need to put the elements in a coherent and meaningful order. The way health services are presented in this book is intended to increase your awareness of the results of health care and how these are achieved. Ultimately, the objective of any health care system is to improve people's health. Hence, a meaningful approach is to describe how health care affects health status.

The approach followed in this book is as follows:

INPUTS → PROCESSES → OUTCOMES

- *Inputs* are the resources needed for health care. Examples include staff, buildings, funds, medical knowledge, drugs, and patients.
- *Processes* describe the use of resources or the activity within the system. Examples include the investigation and treatment of patients, and the referral of patients between facilities. You may also think of organizational processes, such as drug supplies, electronic transmission of information, rationing of care, ways of raising money for the health sector, or paying staff.
- *Outcomes* refer to the change in health status as result of these inputs and processes. These are the results of care, which can be measured in terms of changes in patients' survival or quality of life. But there are many intermediate measures expressing changes in impairment, such as blood sugar levels, body weight or blood pressure, and changes in disability or functional ability, such as mobility or memory.

As you work through the chapters of this book, you will look at the inputs, processes, and outcomes of health services and explore the challenges within each of these categories for the provision of health care.

Before exploring some of these challenges, the next section provides you with an opportunity to look at the factors that have helped shape the health services that exist today.

The role of historical factors in shaping health services

History can provide answers to why there are certain types of health care professionals, why hospitals are located where they are, and why they are organized in a certain style. An analysis of history can also explain the type of carers that are recognized, and those that are not. Many individuals in and outside of health care have been influential in shaping current health services. These include not only clinicians and health care managers but also writers, architects, monarchs, politicians, and philanthropists.

Every country has its own unique historical influences. In some low- and middle-income contexts, there is an influence based on a specific legacy of colonialism (Abel-Smith, 1985). For example, key differences in health services can be seen between countries colonized by the British, French, and Spanish. These influences laid the foundation for the public provision of services in these countries following independence, as services were extended to the wider population. In countries without a colonial history, the private sector has often taken a greater role in service provision.

An analysis of the English health service provides a useful example of how diverse historical factors have helped shape current health services in this context. Nick Black (2012) has identified nine key areas of influence, and these are outlined in Table 1.1.

Table 1.1 Examples from England of the nine historical factors that shape health services

Key influences	Example
Changing conceptions of illness	Changing views on mental health over the last 200 years have influenced the way society, and health services, have responded to mental illness – from seeing it as a dangerous condition requiring custodial confinement, to a treatable illness requiring provision of 'asylums', to treatment in hospitals, and finally to managing patients in the community.
Introduction of new technologies	The introduction of new technologies has shaped how medicine is provided. Before the nineteenth century, care could be provided in simple domestic buildings. With the advent of more advanced technology and more complex surgery, special facilities were needed such as operating theatres. For example, following the discovery of radiation and the introduction of radium to treat cancer, special facilities in hospitals had to be introduced.
Socio-demographic changes	Changing socio-demographic factors have influenced where services are provided. For example, the increasing number of single working people (who had migrated in from rural areas in search of work) in rented accommodation in London by the late nineteenth century had no family to care for them when sick. It was this factor that was a major reason for the establishment of private hospitals.
Social attitudes	Until the mid-nineteenth century, mothers of sick children would not be separated from them, thus precluding admission to hospital. It was Charles Dickens, the writer and social reformer, who managed to persuade parents to let their sick children be cared for in hospital that led to the establishment of children's hospitals.
Religion	In the mid-nineteenth century, religious sisterhoods were responsible for transforming hospitals in London through the organization of the nursing workforce. The religious sisterhood was later to be replaced by the Nightingale (secular) sisterhood.
Finance	Financial factors have influenced the location of hospitals on several occasions. In eighteenth-century London, hospitals were moved away from the city to cheaper land, while in the nineteenth century, hospitals were established near newly built railway stations, which helped to attract more patients (and thus income).
Physical environment	The introduction of trams in London required roads to be widened, which in turn necessitated the demolition of buildings, including hospitals. This led to hospitals having to relocate. Later, the establishment of railways would have a similar impact.
War	Military hospitals have been the site of pioneering innovations in the design and organization of services. The most notable historical example of this is Florence Nightingale's work in the Crimean War (1854–1856), which demonstrated the dangers of hospital-acquired infections and led to measures to reduce risk.
Health care professionals	Health professional teaching needs have influenced the design of hospitals. For instance, wards became increasingly spacious so that senior doctors could be accompanied by ever large numbers of paying medical students, thus enhancing their income.

Knowledge of the influences that have shaped health services in the past can help you recognize factors that are shaping services in the present time. This can assist you to work with and around these factors to address contemporary issues. The next section will help to illustrate this point.

✎ Activity 1.1

Select a country with which you are familiar. Can you identify some historical factors that have helped shape current health services? Try to relate these factors to the nine key factors in Table 1.1.

Feedback

You may have been able to identify some or all of the nine factors above in helping to shape current health services in the context you have chosen. Perhaps some of them are similar to those identified in England, or perhaps you have some very different examples. Take note of your findings and refer back to them as you go through the various chapters in the book.

Factors influencing change and reform in health care

Governments in most countries are concerned about the way health care is provided and reforms are high on the policy agenda. Why have pressures for reform built up over time? In the following article, you will learn how an analysis of the political and economic factors driving these changes can help with understanding these pressures. Arnold Relman, a past editor of the *New England Journal of Medicine*, encapsulated the key concerns of health care policy in an article written at the end of the 1980s (Relman, 1988). Although based on US experience, he describes some of the universal problems of health services. You may find parallels in other countries with which you are familiar.

✎ Activity 1.2

As you read the following edited version of Relman's (1988) article, identify the stages the author describes and make a note of factors that have contributed to growing expenditure. Don't worry about the economic terms, these will be explained later in the book.

When you have read the article, you should be able to address the following:

1   Describe the key features of each of Relman's eras of health care: the era of expansion, the era of cost containment, and the era of assessment and accountability.

2 How did the new funding arrangements, which were introduced in the 1960s, influence development of health services in the USA?
3 Why was cost control alone not considered a successful strategy for managing health services and what criteria does the author suggest for evaluating health services?

Assessment and accountability: the third revolution in medical care

Since the end of World War II the United States has seen two revolutions in its medical care system. It is now on the threshold of a third. The first of these began in the late 1940s and early 1950s and continued through the 1960s. It can be described as the Era of Expansion and was characterized by rapid growth in hospital facilities and the number of physicians, new developments in science and technology, and the extension of insurance coverage to the majority of the population. Medical schools increased and produced an army of new specialists trained in the use of sophisticated technology. The National Institutes of Health poured large resources into basic and clinical research, generating exciting advances that raised public interest and expectations. With the passage of Medicare and Medicaid legislation in 1966, nearly 85 percent of Americans had some form of medical insurance and the goal of universal access to health care seemed close at hand. A final and very important feature of this era was the appearance of investor-owned medical care businesses, mainly hospital chains, which were attracted by the opportunities for profit offered by the open-ended system of insurance payment and the expansion of medical services.

These developments led inevitably to the second revolution, which may be called the Revolt of the Payers or the Era of Cost Containment. More specialists and more technology, many new hospital beds, and a rapidly growing system of health insurance plans that reimburse charges are an explosively inflationary mixture, so it was hardly surprising when per capita medical costs, even after correction for the cost of living, began to rise rapidly. Within two decades after Medicare began, the cost of care had risen from about 4 percent to more than 11 percent of the gross national product, and the trajectory of medical inflation still shows no signs of flattening. At first the third-party payers simply paid the bills, but then employers and the federal government revolted against the costs, and the new era of cost containment began. The result was prospective payment and managed care, as manifested by diagnosis-related groups and health maintenance organizations. Hospitals, formerly in a position to collect whatever they charged, suddenly found themselves facing tougher, monopolistic payers who now were dictating prices. Some states have instituted closely regulated global budgeting for hospitals, and some have established tight controls on new construction. The federal govern-ment has said that it prefers to depend on market competition rather than regulation, but market forces have limited application and dubious ethical standing in health care, and in any case, there is no evidence that competition has been any more successful in keeping costs down than other approaches . . . The chief cause of the cost crisis is not so much the price as the ever increasing volume and intensity of medical services being provided in outpatient settings and hospitals.

Compounding the frustration of the third-party payers in their efforts to control costs is a growing worry about the unknown quality and outcomes of medical services. Furthermore, the discovery of large geographical variations in the incidence of certain services, unaccompanied by any discernible difference in outcome, has led to the suspicion that in many cases we still have much to learn about the indications for a given course of action or the reasons for choosing one procedure over another. It is bad enough, the payers say, to be confronted with uncontrollable medical costs, but the situation becomes intolerable if in addition no one knows what benefits accrue from the services we pay for or the quality of those services. To control costs, without arbitrarily reducing access to care or lowering the quality of care, we will have to know a lot more about the safety, appropriateness and effectiveness of drugs, tests and procedures and the way care is provided by our medical care institutions and profes-sional personnel.

. . . Now, however, we appear to be entering a new era, as a strong new consensus on the need for assessment and accountability seems to be building. At an invitational conference . . . a few months ago, representa-tives from government, private insurers, major corporations, community agencies, and the medical profession met to discuss the problem. There was remarkable unanimity on the conclusion that the time for a new national health care initiative had come. All agreed that to provide a basis for decisions on the future funding and organization of health care, we will have to know more about the variations in performance among institu-tions and medical practitioners and what these may mean. We will also need to know much more about the relative costs, safety, and effective-ness of all the things physicians do or employ in the diagnosis, treatment, and prevention of disease. Armed with these facts, physicians will be in a much stronger position to advise their patients and determine the use of medical resources, payers will be better able to decide what to pay for, and the public will have a better understanding of what is available and what they want.

This theme was sounded by Dr Paul Ellwood in his 1988 Shattuck Lec-ture, published in the Journal a few months ago. Ellwood calls for a major national program of 'outcomes management' by which he means a system linking medical management decisions to new, systematic information about outcomes. He says, correctly I believe, that such a pro-gram 'will not automatically favor a decrease or increase in health care expenditures,' but it will certainly improve the quality and effectiveness of health care and provide a much firmer base for future economic decisions.

. . . To achieve these objectives will require much new financial support and unprecedented cooperation among physicians, government, private insur-ers, and employers. No one should underestimate the size or difficulty of the task. However, the logical necessity of this new initiative seems clear. We can no longer afford to provide health care without knowing more about its successes and failures. The Era of Assessment and Accountability is dawning at last; it is the third and latest – but probably not the last – phase of our efforts to achieve an equitable health care system, of satisfactory quality, at a price we can afford.

From Relman (1988) Assessment and accountability: The third revolution in medical care, *New England Journal of Medicine* 319:1220–2. Adapted with permission from Massachusetts Medical Society.

Feedback

Your responses might be similar to the following:

(1) Relman's three-stage model can be described as follows:

- *Era of expansion, 1940–1960s.* Rapid growth in hospital facilities and doctors. New specialties and new technology raised public expecta-tions. Policies removed the existing financial barriers to health care. New funding arrangements triggered the expansion of health services.
- *Era of cost containment, 1960s–1980s.* The subsequent increase in demand led to a rapid growth of health care expenditure. Often spending grew faster than the national income and policy efforts were focused on cost control. Prospective payment systems started to replace retrospective payment as purchasers of health care began to challenge providers' supremacy.
- *Era of assessment and accountability, 1990s onwards.* Ever-rising costs showed that cost control alone was not effective. Policies of the third era aim to improve the effectiveness and efficiency of ser-vice delivery and use by ensuring that care is appropriate (i.e. the benefits outweigh the costs).

(2) With the introduction of Medicare and Medicaid in 1966, insurance coverage was extended to 85 per cent of the US population, leading to a rapid growth in the number of people with access to health care. As reimbursement for care costs had barely any constraints, the

number of new health service providers increased rapidly as well. Providers were attracted by the prospects of the open-ended system of insurance payments.

(3) A focus on cost control alone could arbitrarily reduce access to care or lower the quality of services provided. For example, denying a new drug on the grounds of higher cost alone might be unwise. Reasons to choose one treatment over another should consider their relative cost-effectiveness. For example, while a new drug might be more expensive than an existing one, it might be worth introducing if it is also more cost-effective. It could provide better value than a cheaper drug, for example, by saving money in other areas of care. (Don't worry if this is unfamiliar to you. You can explore further the economic perspective in other books in the series.)

The essential point here is that health care should be:

- appropriate (effective and safe)
- humane (acceptable to patients)
- equitable (based on a person's need).

Relman argues that the third (and current) era (after expansion and cost containment) aims 'to achieve an equitable health care system, of satisfactory quality, at a price we can afford'.

You may be familiar with other contexts in which the periodization developed by Relman does not apply, but where some of the issues raised by Relman's analysis such as cost containment and accountability are nevertheless pertinent. Therefore, it may be helpful to adapt and utilize the framework in creative and flexible ways.

Understanding contemporary challenges in health services

Having looked at some of the factors leading to current calls for reform, here we present three key issues that may help guide your understanding of the challenges in health services.

First is the relative balance in terms of the influence and control over the decisions around health services between three key roles. These roles are: the health professionals, and in particular the autonomy granted to clinicians within the system; the corporate rationalizers (i.e. the managers, technocrats, and scientists who make decisions at different levels of the system); and lastly, the users of services (patients). You will see that key issues in health services are often a clash between two or more of these groups.

Second is the balance between market forces and 'command and control' approaches in health services. In all countries there will be a mix of state control and market forces influencing how health services are delivered. No country employs one or the other approach in isolation, although some countries come close: in the UK, for example, health services are over 80 per cent publicly funded.

Third is the balance between formal and lay care and who delivers services.

These factors will be explored in more depth in subsequent chapters. You will explore the issues around the role of health professionals; their interaction with each other and with managers; how services are paid for and provided; and the boundaries of lay and formal care. Before going on to look at these areas, the final section of this chapter assesses the contribution that health services research can make to improve the management of services.

The contribution of health services research to management of services

You have seen that there are many questions around how to organize health care and how health services should be managed. In achieving the goal of an equitable health care system, of satisfactory quality, at a price that can be afforded, both research and management play important roles. However, you need to distinguish between health services research (HSR) and investigations that managers perform in the planning and monitoring of health services. Both activities are important, but there are differences, as the examples relating to health centres below illustrate:

1 Researchers aim to make findings that can be *generalized* – for example, in a study to find the optimum distance between health centres, researchers may aim to discover principles that can be applied in various settings.
2 Investigations related to planning and management are of interest in a *particular* situation. An example would be an investigation into where exactly to site health centres in a particular country or an audit to assess the quality of care being provided in a particular hospital.

There is clearly an interactive relationship between management and HSR. As a manager, you would apply results from research and engage in management activities that may give rise to new research.

The scope and contribution of HSR have been outlined in an article by a British researcher, Nick Black (1997). The article introduces the concept of 'environmental turbulence', a useful framework for analysing and understanding the external pressures that any manager will be under.

✎ Activity 1.3

As you read the following edited version of Black's (1997) article, focus on the relationship between management and research and the potential of research to support management. You will see that there are internal and external sources of pressure on health services managers. This activity provides an opportunity to reflect on these pressures and the relevance of HSR in your country.

1   What are the three internal pressures identified by Black?
2   For each of the four main sources of external pressures on management (government, local interests, organizations representing staff, and medical-industrial complex), suggest one example based on your experience in health services.

Health services research: saviour or chimera?

Crises in health services are rarely out of the news. But predictions of impending catastrophe are nothing new (for example, 18th century teaching hospitals felt they were doomed by the rising cost of leeches) and are not confined to countries with highly restricted publicly funded services. Do such crises result from incompetent management or merely indicate the magnitude of the task?

Although there will always be scope for improvements in management, the nature and scale of the task mean that troubles are inevitable. Managers face challenges from both within and outwith their organisations. The internal environment presents three major difficulties. First, health care is highly complex: there are dozens of occupational groups employed in the provision of health care, often competing with one another; complexity also arises because no two patients are identical, which restricts standardised processing; and for many patients, management of their care requires multiple activities to be coordinated. Second, all this complexity is ever changing. And third, unlike many other such organisations, some employees, especially doctors, not only exercise enormous influence on how resources are used, but also have considerable autonomy.

The many external pressures to which health services are subjected have been described as 'environmental turbulence'. Four principal sources of such turbulence can be identified: (1) government, through financial controls, guidance on health-care strategies, and level of social welfare provision; (2) local opinion, local politicians, and consumer organisations;

(3) organisations representing health-care staff, through terms and conditions of service, and training requirements; and (4) the medical-industrial complex, through the promotion of new technologies in which they have commercial interests. All are legitimate stakeholders. It was into this cauldron that health services research (HSR) was introduced in the 1980s. Although research on health services has been undertaken for several decades, it is only in the past 10 years that it has received a huge boost in several industrial countries, including the USA, Canada, and the UK. Why has this happened?

Three influential groups have their reasons and expectations. All payers feel that HSR can help to solve the perennial difficulty of containing increasing costs. Clinicians, smarting from the criticisms of the therapeutic nihilists who had argued that health services had little effect, or even caused more harm than good, believe that research on health care can provide evidence to counter such attacks. The public, whose expectations have rapidly risen with the growth of consumerism, are the third group. These trends have heralded the era of assessment and accountability. But how realistic are these expectations of HSR? Will HSR prove to be a saviour, as many hope and anticipate, or just a chimera, a mere wild fancy or unrealisable dream?

The aim of HSR is to provide unbiased, scientific evidence to influence health services policy at all levels so as to improve the health of the public. It is not a scientific discipline but draws on and uses a wide range of methods from several disciplines, including sociology, statistics, economics, epidemiology, psychology, and history. It also requires input from and an understanding of biology, medicine, nursing, and other clinical areas. HSR challenges the dominant biomedical model in which disease occurs, leading to illness, which is then treated. Although this lies at the heart of the matter, HSR also considers all the other determinants of use of health care. As such, it usually adopts a population perspective, by contrast with the clinical view focusing on individual patients. HSR therefore seeks answers to such questions as: how much health care should we have? How should services be funded? Who should receive services? And, how well are services being provided?

What has HSR ever done for us? To answer this question I have restricted myself to examples in surgery . . .

HSR has identified the value of non-medical aspects of care. My example comes from a much neglected aspect, that of hospital architecture. In a delightful study from the USA, the effect of the view from their hospital window was studied in patients undergoing cholecystectomy. Some were nursed with a view of trees, others with a view of a brick wall. Those with the view of trees required less analgesia, had better psychological adjustment, and had a shorter stay in hospital.

HSR has improved our understanding of who uses services and why. Many factors, apart from the presence of disease, have proved influential, including gender, distance from facilities, patients' knowledge, and clinicians' judgement. Higher rates of appendicectomy in women than in men have long been recognised. Why should this be so? The initial medical response was that females were more likely to develop appendicitis, but no supportive evidence has been forthcoming. The more likely explanations are, first, appendicitis-like symptoms are more common in females, probably arising from ovarian dysfunction. Second, there is evidence in some cultures of young women using the operation to prove their independence. And third, there is widespread availability of surgical services – the gender difference is more pronounced, the higher the overall operation rate in a population.

. . . Surgical rates can also be affected by people's knowledge about the procedure. In the early 1980s there was growing concern in many countries about the high rate of hysterectomies. This was true of Switzerland, where the health office in one canton decided to take action. Rather than try to persuade gynaecologists to be more circumspect in their use of the procedure, they mounted a public information campaign. Two months after the campaign began, the rate started declining, eventually falling by 26%. No change was recorded over this period in a control canton.

The final determinant of use of services I want to consider is clinicians' judgement. In the 1920s in New York City, 1000 11-year-olds had their throats examined. 61% proved to have had their tonsils removed. Of the other 39%, the examining doctor thought about half needed tonsillectomy; the half with healthy tonsils were examined by another doctor, who thought that half of them required surgery. Again, the healthy children were re-examined by yet another doctor who declared that half of them needed the procedure. After four examinations, only 65 of 1000 children would have escaped with their tonsils intact.

Such variation in clinical opinion is not solely a thing of the past. In the 1980s physicians in the USA and the UK were asked to consider several hundred clinical situations and to decide on the appropriateness of coronary surgery. There was a considerable difference: US physicians judged surgery appropriate in more situations than did British physicians (62% vs 41%).

. . . HSR has identified ways of improving the organisation and management of services. One subject that attracts more public and political attention than any other is waiting lists. Despite best endeavours, waiting lists are a permanent feature of health services. Among several reasons for such lists, one is our poor understanding of how waiting lists function. Traditionally, clinicians, managers, and researchers have believed that waiting lists partly reflect a linear queue and partly a mortlake, in which

certain common conditions are sidelined. Attempts to reduce waiting lists which have assumed one or both of these models have often failed. Qualitative study of how waiting lists were being managed revealed that neither model provided a satisfactory account of what was going on. Instead, a list seemed more like a store in which participants – patients, surgeons, clerks, managers – were actively creating, negotiating, and structuring the list. Solutions have to take this concept into account if they are to prove successful.

So is HSR a saviour or a chimera: will it rescue health care from the seemingly impossible dilemmas it faces or will it prove to be no more than an unrealisable dream, a mere wild fancy at the end of the 20th century? HSR has much to contribute, but will never have all the answers. Advocates of rational scientific solutions will therefore have to avoid unjustified claims and engendering unrealistic expectations. HSR can and should only ever be an influence on policy. We must recognise the legitimate role of other forces in shaping health services and seek ways of working with the other parties. In addition, we must not forget that HSR is but a player in a great experiment. We live in a period in which the corporate rationalisers, for whom HSR plays a key part, are challenging the tradition of professional autonomy. Many of us believe such a challenge will lead to a brighter future. But it is only a belief and we may be proved wrong. And we must remember that HSR is the flavour of the decade. But how long will the era of assessment and accountability last? This is but the third revolution in health services. A fourth may be waiting in the wings, so we must take full advantage of the current opportunities.

Reprinted from Black, N. (1997) Health services research: saviour or chimera? *Lancet*, 349:1834–6, with permission from Elsevier.

Feedback

1   Health care is highly complex, which limits the extent to which care can be standardized; this complexity is ever changing; and some employees (notably doctors) exercise enormous influence and have considerable autonomy.
2   You probably found many examples along the lines of those given below.
  • *Government*: almost everywhere governments want managers to meet financial or political targets, for example, to cut public spending or to implement new policies for health services.
  • *Local interests*: local politicians often challenge the views of both managers and central government, as may the local media.
  • *Organizations representing staff*: trade unions fighting for better working conditions and terms of payment; professional organizations influencing training and staffing.

- *Medical-industrial complex*: pharmaceutical companies and other suppliers often promote their products with aggressive marketing and may even resort to bribery.

Although equally important for low-, middle-, and high-income countries, much of HSR to date has been conducted in high-income countries. This is changing, however, with the increasing concerns about health care finance, governments have become more interested in HSR and a number of low- and middle-income countries have started HSR programmes. In countries with academic traditions in public health, HSR is frequently associated with public health schools. But research has also emerged in medical schools and social sciences faculties. You may also find HSR attached to large public institutions like social insurance companies and health care provider organizations. A general concern is that the link between research and management is weak, and it may take a long time for results to disseminate into practice. You need to be aware that much of the success of HSR relies on cooperation with clinicians and managers, yet by its nature HSR tends to challenge established medical knowledge. Successful health services researchers therefore need good political skills as well as strong research abilities.

Summary

Health services are a critical aspect of people's lives and an important area of study. You have seen that an understanding of historical factors that have shaped health services can help in addressing contemporary challenges. You have been introduced to the approach to health services being used in this book. You have learnt that health care reforms are high on the policy agenda in many countries and have explored the factors that help explain how the pressures for current reform have built up over time. Finally, you have looked at the relationship between management and HSR and seen how a research-based approach can contribute to improvement in the quality and management of health services.

References

Abel-Smith, B. (1985) Global perspectives on health service financing, *Social Science and Medicine*, 21 (9): 957–63.

Black, N. (1997) Health services research: saviour or chimera?, *Lancet*, 349 (9068): 1834–6.

Black, N. (2012) *Walking London's Medical History* (2nd edn). London: Hodder Arnold.

Dahlgren, G. and Whitehead, M. (1991) *Policies and Strategies to Promote Social Equity in Health*. Stockholm: Institute for Future Studies.

Moat, K.A. and Abelson, J. (2011) Analysing the influence of institutions on health policy development in Uganda: a case study of the decision to abolish user fees, *African Health Sciences*, 11 (4): 578–86.

Relman, A.S. (1988) Assessment and accountability: the third revolution in medical care, *New England Journal of Medicine*, 319 (18): 1220–2.

World Health Organization Global Health Observatory Data Repository (WHO GHO) (2015) Health expenditure ratios, all countries, selected years – estimates by country. Available at: http://apps.who.int/gho/data/node.main.75?lang=en (accessed 19 April 2016).

Formal and lay care

2

Overview

In Chapter 1 you were introduced to the distinction between formal and lay (informal) care and to the idea that health care is delivered at different levels. In this chapter you will study the boundaries of formal care and lay care in more detail and how lay care contributes to formal care at each level of care. Finally, you will look at the different attitudes of the formal sector towards lay care.

Learning objectives

After working through this chapter, you will be able to:

- outline the different levels at which health care is provided
- outline the difference between formal care and lay care
- understand the contribution of lay care to wider formal care at different levels
- understand the different viewpoints on lay care by the formal sector

Key terms

Formal care: Care provided by trained, paid professionals usually in a formal setting.

Lay care: Care provided by lay people who have received no formal training and are not paid. It includes self-care and care provided by relatives, friends, and self-help groups.

Primary care: Formal care that is the first point of contact for people. It is usually general rather than specialized and provided in the community.

Secondary care: Specialized care that often can only be accessed by being referred by a primary care worker. It is usually provided in local hospitals.

> **Self-help groups:** Groups of unpaid, self-taught people that offer solutions to health problems in a lay setting, based on mutual support between persons experiencing similar conditions.
>
> **Tertiary care:** Highly specialized care that often can only be accessed by referral from secondary care. It is usually provided in national or regional hospitals.

Levels of health care

As you saw in Chapter 1, health care covers a wide range of activities, including those relating to cure, prevention, and care. In addition to the breadth of activities, there are also different *levels* of care. In the provision of health care, we can distinguish three levels of care:

- *Primary care*: this is the first point of contact with the population and may be provided within the community through outreach or in a small health facility at community level. The service provided is usually general and may cover a wide range of activities such as immunization, antenatal care, monitoring of conditions, and minor surgery. Patients requiring more specialist care may be referred to the secondary or tertiary level. Care is mostly provided by nurses and general practitioners. In some countries, community workers may provide basic curative care or preventative activities at this level.
- *Secondary care*: this is care that is often accessed by referral from the primary level. It is more specialized in nature. Examples of care at this level include orthopaedic surgery or psychiatry. Care is provided in a range of health care facility settings, often small hospitals, depending on the context.
- *Tertiary care*: this is highly specialized care that is often accessed by referral from the secondary level, though in some cases this link is by-passed and people are referred direct from the primary level. Tertiary care is usually provided in large hospitals at regional or national level, and by highly specialized professional staff. Care at this level may include such diverse activities as cardiac surgery or the provision of secure accommodation for offenders with mental health conditions.

Activity 2.1

Like many definitions, the definitions of level of care are not watertight and exceptions exist. Can you suggest some health care activities that do not fit these definitions?

Figure 2.1 provides a representation of the levels of care. As you can see, lay care is shown as underpinning the three levels of care. However, as you will now explore, there is an important role for lay care at each of the levels of care.

Lay versus formal care

You may be wondering why it is important to study the relationship between formal and lay care. In fact, there are several important reasons. In the first instance, most health care, estimated to be 80 per cent of all care, is provided by people with no formal training and often in a voluntary capacity. Lay care therefore makes a substantial contribution to overall care. Second, the involvement of lay care can have an important impact on formal care, and studying lay care can help your understanding of care-seeking behaviour

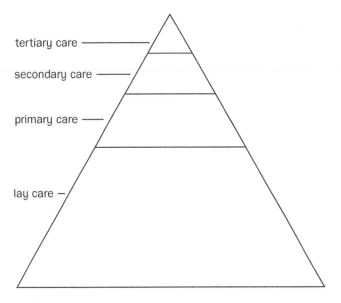

Figure 2.1 Formal and lay care

more broadly. Finally, an understanding of a lay perspective is an essential aspect of ensuring community participation and promoting a sense of ownership of local health services. This aspect is explored further in Chapter 8. Lay care can take a number of forms:

- *Providing information and advice*: this may be advice on what course of action to take or information on certain conditions. For example, in some countries voluntary health workers play a role in providing health information on infant feeding, or encouraging the uptake of services such as vaccination or antenatal care. The involvement of lay workers can have a significant positive impact on the uptake of formal services.
- *Emotional support*: this may cover a number of situations. It may include the provision of support following an adverse life event such as a bereavement, which can undermine a person's health. It might mean supporting someone to stop a habit that is detrimental to their health, such as smoking. It may also be helping someone recuperate after an illness, or providing someone with ongoing support for a chronic condition.
- *Practical assistance*: this covers a number of ways of providing support for health care such as monitoring symptoms, helping with medications, or providing support for washing and eating. In some situations, this care may come very close to what is viewed as formal care (Clark et al., 2008).

It is easy to see that there is considerable blurring of the boundaries between formal and lay care. To help distinguish between the sectors, a number of criteria have been developed. However, you may find that, even when applying these criteria, it is sometimes difficult to separate the boundaries between the two types of care. Existing criteria cover the following:

- *The setting*: formal care usually takes place in a recognized setting, such as a GP's surgery or a health centre, while lay care usually takes place in an informal setting, such as a person's home. However, it is possible to think of exceptions to both these situations. For instance, the role of voluntary staff in providing support in hospitals and hospices.
- *The training (or level of skill involved)*: those involved in formal care usually receive formal training that receives some form of recognition. Lay care workers, in contrast, usually receive no or very limited training that is not officially recognized. However, this is not always the case. In some contexts, voluntary community workers may undergo a formal training course, albeit of short duration and at a basic level. At the end of this training, a certificate may be presented, although this may only be recognized in the particular context in which it has been awarded.
- *The rewards*: formal carers are paid in money or in kind, while lay care workers are usually not. However, in some cases community workers may receive a small payment or payment in kind. This introduces another 'grey area' when trying to distinguish between the different types of care.

Activity 2.2

The following activity is designed to help you reflect on the extent of lay care in practice, as well as who provides it.

1   Choose a country with which you are familiar. Write down examples of lay care that exist in that country. Bear in mind that lay care covers a wide range of activities, including health promotion, nursing, diagnosis, and treatment. What factors do you think determine the role of lay care in the country you have chosen?
2   Think of traditional healers or alternative therapists in the country you have chosen. According to the criteria outlined above, are they formal or lay carers?
3   In the country you have chosen, which members of the family would be most likely to care for an elderly or disabled relative?

Feedback

1   You probably had no difficulty in finding a wide range of examples of lay care. You may have had some difficulty in deciding whether some particular candidates were lay or formal carers. The distinction can sometimes be difficult. Several factors determine the role of lay care: the level of economic development, views about the relative responsibilities of individuals and the state, cultural and religious beliefs, family structure (including geographical dispersion of families), and the power of the formal carers.
2   You should have identified traditional healers or alternative therapists as formal carers. They have usually received some formal training and are usually paid.
3   Mostly, women provide lay care and this appears to be a universal phenomenon.

The extent of lay care

Compared with what is known about formal care, there is little information available on the extent of lay care, either from studies or routine records. It is therefore hard to get a clear picture of the full extent of lay practice and its contribution to overall health services. However, where studies are available, they show that the largest proportion of care is delivered as lay care. This includes self-care and care provided by family members. This is true for a range of country contexts. The amount of time spent caring may be considerable. One study of caregivers of people with motor neurone disease estimated that the amount of time spent in lay care is as much as 10 hours per day, sometimes longer. This level of care was found in more than 30 per cent of the sample (Peters et al., 2012).

In the UK, one in eight adults cares for someone else to some extent. This doesn't take into account routine parenting such as caring for a sick child. Much of this activity is social care (washing, feeding, dressing), although an increasing number of carers are also assisting with the administration of formal health care, such as giving intravenous drugs (Kirk and Glendinning, 1998; Pickard and Glendinning, 2002).

It has been shown that lay care is most often provided by females rather than males, and this remains the case even when both sexes are employed. In one study looking at the care provided to a relative with a disability, women on average spent three hours per day providing care, while men spent just 13 minutes doing so (Nissel and Bonnerjea, 1982). Another study found that the responsibility for staying at home with a sick child was heavily weighted towards the mother (74 per cent) rather than the father (40 per cent), even though both parents were working (Smith and Schaeffer, 2012). This is the case even when the parents are both doctors: a study of 400 couples where both partners worked full-time as a doctor found that 80 per cent of the men viewed it to be the woman's responsibility to care for the child when sick (Elston, 1980).

Most people make use of formal and lay care, and learn from an early age how to determine which is appropriate for which situation. Think for a moment about what you would do if you woke with abdominal pain. If it was mild, you might decide to do nothing and see if the pain passes. If it persisted, you might self-medicate with some medicine available 'over the counter' from a shop or consult a friend or family member. If it still continued, you might refer yourself to a formal carer, such as a doctor. The decision about which sector to use is not fixed but will vary with the condition. It will also depend on the services available, which in turn will be determined by various contextual factors such as the level of financing for health care.

An article by Roland Msiska and colleagues (1997) describes the diversity of options for people living in Zambia who are suffering from a sexually transmitted disease (STD). The researchers were attempting to find out what determined people's choices.

✎ Activity 2.3

As you read the following, edited version of Msiska and colleagues' (1997) article, make notes on (1) the care options available, and (2) the factors that influenced people's decisions to use either lay or formal care.

Understanding lay perspectives: care options for STD treatment in Lusaka, Zambia

Introduction

Studies conducted in the developing and developed world have identified several determinants for health care-seeking behaviour patterns for various types of illness. These include type and severity of symptoms, the course of illness, sick role, perception regarding cause of illness, age, sex, education and economic status, social cost, social networking and lay referral mechanisms, availability of the service and their opinion of the efficacy of therapeutic options. These factors interact in a complex and diverse manner, and vary in their direction and power of influence on the behaviour of individuals or communities.

The objective of this study was to determine lay persons' perspectives in care-seeking behaviour patterns for STD in selected sub-populations in Lusaka.

Methods

A combination of 20 unstructured interviews, 10 focus group discussions (FGDs) and four STD illness simulations were performed in purposively selected sub-populations with a varied age and sex mix in order to obtain information on health care-seeking behaviour patterns.

. . . In general, the problem of HIV/AIDS was perceived as a greater and far more serious threat than other STDs and little linkage was recognized between the two conditions. The commonest STDs identified were syphilis (kaswende), gonorrhoea ('leakage' or pus) and chancroid (bola bola), all of which were considered treatable with 'proper medicine'. Of interest is the fact that in spite of this knowledge, people believed that traditional medicine was still relevant in ensuring a satisfactory outcome in addition to hospital treatment. Traditional medicine is usually obtained from friends or older men and women who are conversant in the treatment of STDs.

Participants preferred private facilities to public health facilities – this includes private general practitioners, private chemists, street vendors and market stalls. Street and market vendors had an array of medicines which they prescribed according to the clients' description of the STD. The reasons for not wanting to use public health institutions for STD treatment were mainly the social costs and 'inconvenience' associated with hospitals and clinics rather than economic constraints (after all, as participants indicated, in Lusaka the GPs are far more expensive than the public health institutions). According to the clients, the set-up of the STD service at the University Teaching Hospital did not encourage them to go there because it was too cumbersome and left people vulnerable to exposure and embarrassment. For example, a client has to describe his/her symptoms to several health workers (including guards controlling the queues!) before reaching the right clinic. Derogatory remarks by staff, especially those attributing STD to lack of or loose morals, also contributed to the reluctance to attend the service. Compulsory partner attendance as a pre-condition to treatment also discouraged clients. In contrast to the public health institutions, GPs and street vendors tended to provide a quick 'no-questions-asked' service that appealed to and was approved by clients.

A total of four STD case simulations were carried out in private pharmacies. The results indicate that the sale of antibiotics for STDs has become a roaring and lucrative business in the compounds. Little or no information is provided to the buyer on the use of the drugs or on the type of drug being given. Of all the four pharmacies visited, only one refused to sell antibiotics without a doctor's prescription. The street vendors sold all kinds of antibiotics with little regard for packaging, duration or instructions for use. The amount of drug sold depended on the amount of money the client had.

Discussion

Patterns for STD care

Earlier studies in Lusaka revealed that options open to the sick 'are of bewildering complexity. They include . . . consultations with relatives, with white, Indian or fellow African employees of diverse tribal and linguistic origins; with neighbours and friends . . . Western doctors' (Frankenberg and Leeson, 1976). The 10 focus group discussions and the 20 unstructured interviews in the bars confirm the diversity and complex nature of the care options, which in the case of STD include an array of options. These include self-medication, traditional healers, medicines sold in the markets and streets, as well as injections administered in the compounds. Private clinics, health centres and hospitals also provide a service, though the latter are perceived by clients to provide a less satisfactory service. As for drugs used in the treatment of STDs, these were widely available in the markets, stores and pharmacies. These antibiotics were being prescribed without any sort of regulatory framework and in circumstances that posed danger and doubt for the patient's successful treatment. This has the potential to cause drug resistance, thus further complicating the prevention of STD in Zambia.

Self-care

The term 'self-care' has diverse interpretations. The definition used in this study is that of Levin in which he describes self-care as 'a process by which people function on their own behalf in health promotion and prevention and in disease detection and treatment at the level of the primary resource in the health care system' (Levin, 1981). This is further elaborated by John Fry into four elements of self-care, namely: health maintenance, self-medication, self-treatment, and participation in professional care. In all the 10 focus groups and 20 unstructured interviews, self-care was a predominant option in dealing with STDs. Self-care is particularly important in STDs due to the shame and stigma and social cost attached to the management of the illness.

Although there is little consistency in the definition of self-care among researchers, studies have shown as high as 65–85 per cent of health care is self-care. In the absence of studies on the quality of self-care that STD patients are providing for themselves, there is a potential danger of the emergence of resistant strains of STD organisms, of partially treated STDs and hence of increased complications. On the other hand, self-care provides an opportunity for universal coverage for STD treatment in a resource-constrained environment such as Zambia. In the words of Levin 'strengthening self-care . . . seems to represent a basic thrust towards a more adequate, more accessible, more dignified, and possibly more effective mode of using health resources, irrespective of the particular health delivery or financing system or, for that matter, political environment'. Strengthening self-care in Zambia provides an opportunity for the full partnership of lay persons and professionals in health care, consistent with the overall thrust of the health reform.

Factors influencing care-seeking behaviour

The factors identified as influencing care-seeking behaviour are: lay referral mechanisms, social cost, availability of care options, economic factors, beliefs, stigma and quality of care as perceived by the users.

Lay referral mechanisms

As may be expected for an illness such as STD, exchange of information on STDs occurred within age and sex groups. Stigma and social cost associated with STDs made it difficult for students to consult elders on how to manage STDs once afflicted. Peer consultation was identified as the predominant approach among the students once infected with STDs.

Social cost

Social cost refers to 'the restructuring of personal relationships, customary exchange patterns and friendship ties that often accompany innovation'. The evidence from this study suggests that social cost is higher for female STD patients than male patients, in that, although women preferred to be examined by female staff, they were still being examined by men. The majority of clinical officers in Zambia are male and these are usually the front-line in the screening of STD patients.

Other aspects of social cost identified by all groups included being required to bring partners before STD treatment would be provided and the lack of privacy. The process of reducing social cost is reflected by the patients' preference for traditional healers rather than medical staff. The female participants observed that ' ... traditional healers would not request you to undress before providing you with treatment or insist that you need to bring a partner before giving one treatment'. Traditional healers rarely asked 'too many questions', as one participant said.

Expression of stigma

STD in the participating communities is highly stigmatized; it is associated with the use of labels such as fimbusu (literally translated as toilets) and hule (prostitutes). In all focus groups these terms were mainly used in relation to women suffering from STD, not men. Terms used to describe men suffering from STD had less offensive labelling, for example, kubukinsa, which in literal translation means having an accident. In one focus group, females indicated that suffering from an STD was worse than having a child out of wedlock! This influences not only the recognition of symptoms but also the process of consultation and care-seeking patterns.

Gender

As stated above, social cost is highest for female STD patients since the examining doctors tend to be male. Women were also disadvantaged by the requirement to bring partners as a condition of receiving treatment.

Staff attitudes and the location of STD clinics made it difficult for patients to access the health facilities within the area studied. Social culture expectations of women make this process particularly difficult for them.

Problems associated with use of government health centres and hospitals

In order to understand what is lacking in professional care from the groups' perspective, all groups were asked what they thought were the difficulties involved in obtaining treatment for STDs at government health centres and hospitals. The following emerged as problems: shortage of drugs, lack of privacy, long queues, being examined by a member of the opposite sex, high medical fees, demanding the attendance of the partner before provision of treatment. Focus group participants were unanimous in their opinion that the shortage of drugs was a creation of the health centre medical staff. This was confirmed, in their view, by the fact that some medical staff were 'selling' them drugs for STD treatment in the compounds.

Reprinted from Msiska, R., Nangawe, E., Mulenga, D., Sichone, M., Kamanga, J. and Kwapa, P. (1997) Understanding lay perspectives: care options for STD treatment in Lusaka, Zambia, *Health Policy and Planning*, 12 (3): 248–52, with permission from Oxford University Press.

The changing nature of lay care

Many commentators have noted that the nature of lay care is changing. Developments in the socio-economic circumstances of populations and a weakening of kinship obligations are having an impact on the availability of lay care in many countries. In particular, the capacity for lay care is reducing as more women enter employment. At the same time, greater geographical mobility is separating family members, and care is increasingly being confined to the nuclear family.

The result is that larger numbers of people, in particular older people, are living alone without access to lay care. This phenomenon is having an effect on the provision of health services because, in the absence of lay care, an increasing number of older people are in need of formal care. In the UK, older people remain in hospital longer than is considered absolutely necessary, as their discharge from hospital is delayed due to insufficient care for them at home or in the community. This is contributing to an additional pressure on the availability of hospital beds (Glasby et al., 2006).

However, despite these changes, it is important to be aware that throughout the world there remains a willingness to care for the older members of society on the part of families, and that most of the care is still provided by lay carers.

Attitudes towards lay care by formal care workers

The relationship between formal care workers and lay care is important if the two sectors are to work constructively together and enhance each other's contribution to overall care. Over the last few decades, there have been a variety of responses to the emergence of a more vociferous and confident lay sector. Three different responses can be identified:

1 A range of care-related activities ought only to be provided by trained formal carers with adequate knowledge and training. Therefore, formal care needs to expand to cover care provided by lay carers. This viewpoint

is perhaps linked to a concern that a dynamic lay care sector could be used to cut spending on formal care.

2 Lay carers are capable of being trained by formal carers to carry out specific tasks that are at the discretion of formal care providers. The extent of lay care is thus determined and 'granted' by formal carers.

3 Lay care workers should be encouraged and supported by formal care workers. Given the overwhelming need for care in the population, the lay sector can provide much-needed support to the formal sector. In this view, the independence of lay carers is encouraged rather than restricted and controlled. Lay contributions are seen as an opportunity to support the formal sector, rather than a threat.

✎ Activity 2.4

Think of the provision of services in a country with which you are familiar. How does lay care currently support the formal sector? Is the role of lay care changing in this context? Why is this the case and what do you think are the implications?

Feedback

Whatever context you have chosen, you will likely have identified the important role that lay care is playing in the provision of health services, whether this is through special cadres of lay staff, or the role played by many people, often women, in supporting care in the home or community. You may have noticed that this role is changing. Perhaps there has been a rise in the need for care for older people in your chosen context; perhaps the role that has been traditionally played by women in providing care is under threat from rising opportunities for employment for women outside the home. Perhaps you see implications of this from stories in the media or personal experience.

Summary

Health care is provided at different levels – primary, secondary, and tertiary – and lay care can support formal care at each level. A recognition of the distinction between formal and lay care is important for understanding the scope of health care. The major part of care is provided by the lay sector in an informal setting and is unpaid. Lay care is thus a major determinant of the amount of formal care consumed. Lay care can take a range of different forms: individual self-care, care within families and social networks, and self-help groups. You have explored the key factors that are changing the availability of lay care and what this means for formal care.

You have looked at the different attitudes of the formal sector towards lay care, and the implications of these for support to lay care.

The remainder of the book is devoted to formal care. The following chapters will explore formal care in more detail and you will look at how services are organized in terms of the inputs (e.g. health staff, financing, medical knowledge), the processes or activities to provide care (e.g. immunization, operations), the processes to ensure the quality of care (e.g. quality assessment and quality improvement), and finally, the outcomes that result (e.g. mortality, morbidity, disability and quality of life) (Donabedian, 1988, 2003).

References

Clark, A.M., Reid, M.E., Morrison, C.E., Capewell, S., Murdoch, D.L. and McMurray, J.J. (2008) The complex nature of informal care in home-based heart failure management, *Journal of Advanced Nursing*, 61 (4): 373–83.

Donabedian, A. (1988) The quality of care: how can it be assessed?, *Journal of the American Medical Association*, 260 (12): 1743–7.

Donabedian, A. (2003) *An Introduction to Quality Assurance in Health Care*. Oxford: Oxford University Press.

Elston, M.A. (1980) Medicine: half of our future doctors?, in R. Silverstone and A. Ward (eds) *Careers of Professional Women*. London: Croom Helm.

Frankenberg, R. and Leeson, J. (1976) Disease, illness and sickness: social aspects of the choice of healer in a Lusaka urban community, in J.B. London (ed.) *Social Anthropology and Medicine*. New York: Academic Press.

Glasby, J., Littlechild, R. and Pryce, K. (2006) All dressed up but nowhere to go? Delayed hospital discharges and older people, *Journal of Health Services Research and Policy*, 11 (1): 52–8.

Kirk, S. and Glendinning, C. (1998) Trends in community care and patient participation: implications for the roles of informal carers and community nurses in the United Kingdom, *Journal of Advanced Nursing*, 28 (2): 370–81.

Levin, L.S. (1981) Self-care in health: potentials and pitfalls, *World Health Forum*, 2: 177–84.

Msiska, R., Nangawe, E., Mulenga, D., Sichone, M., Kamanga, J. and Kwapa, P. (1997) Understanding lay perspectives: care options for STD treatment in Lusaka, Zambia, *Health Policy and Planning*, 12 (3): 248–52.

Nissel, M. and Bonnerjea, L. (1982) *Family Care of the Handicapped Elderly: Who pays?*, Paper #602. London: Policy Studies Institute.

Peters, M., Fitzpatrick, R., Doll, H., Playford, E.D. and Jenkinson, C. (2012) The impact of perceived lack of support provided by health and social care services to caregivers of people with motor neurone disease, *Amyotrophic Lateral Sclerosis*, 13 (2): 223–8.

Pickard, S. and Glendinning, C. (2002) Comparing and contrasting the role of family carers and nurses in the domestic health care of frail older people, *Health and Social Care in the Community*, 10 (3): 144–50.

Smith, K. and Schaeffer, A. (2012) *Who Cares for the Sick Kids? Parents' access to paid time to care for a sick child*. Durham, NH: Carsey Institute, University of New Hampshire [online].

SECTION 2

Inputs to health care

Diseases and medical knowledge 3

Overview

This chapter discusses one of the key aspects of health care, namely an understanding of the concepts of disease and medical knowledge. In this chapter, you will learn what is meant by disease and how ideas of disease change over time and place. You will explore how cultural factors influence medical knowledge and how this contributes to an understanding of the international differences between health services. Finally, you will look at the issue of the medicalization of conditions and what this means for health services.

Learning objectives

After working through this chapter, you will be able to:

- outline the concept of 'disease' and describe how it relates to social and cultural factors
- describe how medical knowledge is generated and how categories of diseases arise
- analyse the relationship between culture and medicine and show how cultural factors affect international comparisons
- understand what is meant by the 'medicalization' of conditions and the impact of this on health services

Key terms

Culture: The values, beliefs, and attitudes associated with a social system.

Disease: A condition, which, judged by the prevailing culture, is painful or disabling and deviates from either the statistical norm or from some idealized status.

Diseases: Patterns of factors (symptoms, signs) that occur in many people in more or less the same way.

Felt need: A person's subjective assessment of their need (self-assessment).

Iatrogenesis: Disease or harm resulting from health care interventions.

Medicalization: The preference for defining problems as 'medical' and thus subject to the involvement of medical practitioners (also referred to as medical imperialism).

Normative need: A professional assessment of a person's need based on objective measures (professional or biomedical assessment).

Pathological: Form or function that is deemed to be abnormal.

Physiological: Bodily function (such as breathing) that is deemed to be 'normal'.

Differences between objective and subjective explanations of disease

Health services are often described and studied in terms of disease groups or patients' groups, as though these categories are unproblematic. However, this is not necessarily the case. For example, it is important to consider two questions: what is 'disease'?, and what are 'diseases'? You may think this to be straightforward: disease is what doctors define to be ill health. But as you will explore in this section, the concept of 'disease' is more complex and is fundamental to an understanding of health services.

Let us start by defining disease. You could define disease as the absence of health, and health as the absence of disease. However, these are circular definitions based on the absence of the other, and do not help you get to an understanding of what is meant by 'disease'. To do this you need to look at the two approaches to defining disease: self-assessment and professional assessment.

Self-assessment relates to how a person feels about their own health. This is necessarily subjective. It is an assessment of 'felt need' and an indication of a person's 'need for health'. This assessment of health will vary from person to person. At one extreme, there are the 'stoics' who will tolerate more pain or discomfort than others; at the other extreme, there are the 'hypochondriacs', who will complain about the slightest problem. Most people lie somewhere in the continuum between these two extremes, and will be more or less stoical or prone to hypochondria. This will influence the person's 'felt need'. In addition, people without a medical background may not always distinguish between symptoms of a disease and symptoms that are part of the normal physiological processes in life, such as pregnancy and teething. This may also impact on their 'felt need'.

Professional or biomedical assessment relates to the use of objective, scientific definitions of illness and is often based on statistical probability definitions of illness. Biomedical observation uses signs and test results to define disease. Professional definitions may also include whether a cost-effective treatment is available. In this sense, the definition is based on a person's 'need for health care'. It is sometimes referred to as 'normative need'. Despite the sophisticated tools available to test for disease, it may still be difficult for a professional to judge whether disease is present or not. This is because many measures are 'continuous' (on a continuum) rather than 'dichotomous' (present or absent), and a judgement about whether a person has a disease still has to be made. For example, the level of iron in the blood at which anaemia is diagnosed.

Felt need and normative need may differ in their assessment of disease for many reasons, as you will explore in the following sections. The extract below provides an opportunity to think about some of these reasons.

✎ Activity 3.1

In 1954, Lester King, an American doctor, explored the distinction between subjective and objective definitions of disease. King defined disease as: 'the aggregate state of those conditions, which, judged by the prevailing culture, are deemed painful or disabling and which at the same time deviate from either the statistical norm or from some idealized status'. As you read the following extract from his article, 'What is disease?', write down an example for each of the following statements:

1 Disease varies with cultural context.
2 Some painful conditions are not considered a disease.
3 There is deviance from a statistical norm that is not deemed pathological.
4 A deviance from an idealized state could be a disease, even though it doesn't deviate from the statistical norm.

What is disease?

As illustrating the confusion surrounding the notion of disease, I recall a very precise young physician who asked me what our laboratory considered the normal hemoglobin level of the blood (with the particular technique we used). When I answered, '12 to 16 grams, more or less,' he was very puzzled. Most laboratories, he pointed out, called 15 grams normal, or perhaps 14.5. He wanted to know how, if my norm was so broad and vague, he could possibly tell whether a patient suffered from anemia, or how much anemia. I agreed that he had quite a problem on his hands, and that it is a very difficult thing to tell. So difficult, in fact, that trying to be too precise is actually misleading, inaccurate, stultifying to thought, and philosophically very unsound.

He wanted to know why I didn't take one hundred or so normal individuals, determine their hemoglobin by our method, and use the resulting figure as the normal value for our method. This, I agreed, was a splendid idea. But how were we to pick out the normals? The obvious answer is, just take one or two hundred healthy people, free of disease . . . But that is exactly the difficulty. We think health as freedom from disease, and disease as an aberration from health. This is traveling in circles, getting us nowhere.

. . . One way of determining health is by this subjective report. The man who says, 'I feel just fine,' may consider himself entirely sound. Conversely, he who complains of feeling 'terrible' may think of himself as seriously ill. These subjective impressions are essential, and highly significant, but they are not entirely reliable. Here we come up against the distinction between what 'seems' and what 'really is,' between 'appearance' and 'reality.' We are all familiar with the man who had periodic routine examinations, who passed all tests, who felt subjectively fine, and who suddenly dropped dead. Or the man with no complaints at all but, cajoled into a routine chest x-ray, found he has a symptomless cancer. In such cases the individual 'seemed' healthy, subjectively he felt healthy, but 'really' he wasn't.

To understand health or disease we must have some objective measurements in addition to the introspective account. If we can weigh or measure something, then we have a little more confidence, and we feel more firmly grounded in objective reality. And there is no end of different features that we can thus quantitate. With the help of measurements and statistical analysis we can get a very whole picture of what exists and in what distribution, and, moreover, what we may reasonably expect in the future. But ordinarily statistics alone cannot label any part of the data as 'diseased.' When we apply statistical methods we already have in mind the idea of health. We exert selection on the cases we study. Thus, to find the 'normal' blood sugar level we eliminate known diabetics. And the basal metabolic rate, in health, we determine after omitting known thyroid disease.

In spite of the circularity, the concepts of health and disease belong together. There are certain factors which are important for defining and distinguishing them. One is the subjective report, which is of only moderate reliability. The sense of well-being frequently correlates with what we mean by health, but the correlation is not high. Certainly a sense of well-being does not preclude the prevalence of disease, while the absence of such subjective feeling does not indicate disease.

Another important factor is the statistical distribution, quite independent of any subjective report. Let us imagine, for example, a statistical study of body temperature, on completely random samples. We would find an overwhelming majority of individuals within a narrow band, between 98 and 99° F. However, a very small percentage will show much higher figures, such as 102°, 101°, or 105°, or more. These individuals who depart from the norm, are by definition abnormal. This deviation, by itself, does not make them diseased. Thus, persons with an intelligence quotient of 180, or with the ability to run 100 yards in 9.4 seconds, are also highly abnormal. However, when a deviation is tied up with malaise, pain, or death, or is intimately associated with conditions which lead to disability or death, then the abnormality forms part of disease.

Statistical norms, even when correlated with malaise, can furnish only a part of the total picture. For example, statistics can establish the normal body temperature and, by correlation with malaise, pain, or death, the desirable body temperature. But in the matter of, say, dentition, the statistical norm does not define the healthy or the desirable. Very few native Americans possess thirty-two intact, well-aligned teeth. Yet when we speak of sound or healthy dentition we have in mind the ideal of thirty-two intact, well-aligned teeth. In this case it is deviation from the ideal which constitutes disease, not deviation from a statistical norm.

These ideals stem from two sources. One is concrete observation. Nothing can serve as a model of health unless it has been an observed characteristic or feature. And second, any such feature must be an object of general desire, possessing value which appeals to the mass of the population. One person might desire to be eight feet tall, yet the majority of people do not. The ideals of height, of weight, of bust measurement, or head size, that is, the range which the majority desires, vary from one nation or tribe to another, and from one generation to another. Changes in diet, for example, can in a few generations change the ideals in regard to stature. But at the present time a height of eight feet is not a matter of general craving.

. . . Disease lies in the realm of pain, discomfort, or death. There are, however, many examples of pain and discomfort which we cannot so designate. A teething infant or a woman in childbirth, are suffering pain. We may try to relieve this pain, but we do not think of teething or childbirth as diseases. We call them normal functions. To be a healthy infant is to go through a period of teething. We conclude that discomfort which constantly attends a normal desirable function and is intimately or essentially bound up with that desirable function, is not in the realm of disease.

It follows that our concepts of disease are very closely related to our values. Frequently our values may be severely determined by convention. China, for example, did not regard as diseased those upper-class women whose feet were bound, and who thereby suffered pain and diminution in function. Our contemporary culture takes a different view which means that our conventions and values of health are different from the Chinese. In most of our western civilization the seeing of visions we consider a sign of a diseased state. But in some epochs of our civilization the seer of visions was a leader in the community, receiving special honor because of his unusual endowment. Certainly the egregious and unusual, the literally abnormal, represent disease only if judged by indigenous cultural values. Convention plays a very important part in shaping our values. And the quantity of our knowledge plays a very important part in shaping our conventions.

Disease is the aggregate of those conditions which, judged by the prevailing culture, are deemed painful, or disabling, and which, at the same time, deviate from either the statistical norm or from some idealized status. Health, the opposite, is the state of well-being conforming to the ideals of the prevailing culture, or to the statistical norm. The ideal itself is derived in part from the statistical norm, and in part from the abnormal which seems particularly desirable.

Feedback

1 You may have thought of foot binding in traditional Chinese society or low blood pressure, considered a disease in Germany but elsewhere not.
2 Teething, childbirth.
3 Obviously a number of biomedical parameters vary without being related to pathology, for example, a high blood sugar level after a meal does not imply diabetes.
4 Dental health in a population of elderly people – although the number of teeth lost does not deviate from the statistical norm (as all in that age group have fewer teeth), the condition deviates from the idealized state.

Other examples of how the boundary between being healthy and being diseased may vary between places and over time include:

* *Malaria*: in Europe, any person with a parasitaemia (presence of malaria parasites in the blood) would be treated, whereas in tropical endemic areas where 60 per cent of the population may have a parasitaemia but no symptoms, only persons with manifest disease would be treated.
* *Dyslexia*: has been recognized as a diseased state in recent years whereas previously it was not.

From the examples, you can see that disease is not just a biomedical issue but also a 'social construct'. Our understanding and acceptance of ill health can be constructed by different social factors, including how ill health is supported. This latter point is illustrated by data on retirement rates for ill health in the UK during the 1990s. These rates show large variation across different professions, which can be correlated with the package of entitlements to benefits. There is also large variation in regional rates for ill health. These data support the view that something other than the natural variation of ill health or exposure to disease-causing factors is influencing retirement rates.

How do disease categories arise?

Having explored the concept of disease, let us now look at the different ways in which diseases are categorized. This is important to build up a consistent picture of which diseases are impacting on people's health, and the implications of this for health services.

Medical knowledge is based on categorizing states of ill health into discrete diseases. Diseases are patterns of factors (symptoms, signs) that occur in many people in more or less the same way. These categories occur for a number of reasons and you need to be aware that just as the notion of disease can change, so can the categorization of diseases. Studying these changes can help you understand the complex world of disease categorization. Changes occur for five reasons:

1 Real changes (new diseases)
2 Changes in name
3 Sub-division of categories
4 Changes in recognition of abnormal
5 Uncovering previously rare conditions.

Real changes can occur when a new disease emerges or a disease disappears. Examples of newly emergent diseases include HIV/AIDS and new variant Creutzfeldt-Jacob disease. Diseases that have disappeared include: sweating sickness (English Sweat), which occurred in five epidemics between 1486 and 1551 and then disappeared; endemic Tyrolean infantile cirrhosis, which lasted from 1900 to 1974; and encephalitis lethargica, which appeared in Europe and North America between 1919 and 1926 (and which may be reappearing in the twenty-first century).

Often the change is in name only. Coronary heart disease is a good example. Many different names were used for the same disease before the name coronary heart disease was created (Stehbens, 1987). Another example is glue ear (otitis media with effusion). The name for this same condition has changed more than 50 times since the nineteenth century (Black, 1984).

Sometimes change occurs because there is a sub-division of categories for a disease, based on a better understanding of the disease. This is a common phenomenon with the progress of medical knowledge. For example, diabetes was initially split into *diabetes insipidus* and *diabetes mellitus* on the basis of the appearance and taste of a patient's urine. The latter was then divided into type 1 and type 2 on the basis of the distinction of the problem as a failure of the person to create insulin or a failure of the body to respond to insulin. More recently, advances in molecular biology have contributed to an understanding of the further various sub-categories of the different types of diabetes.

Another example of sub-categories is childhood diarrhoea in Bangladesh. Local people recognize four types of diarrhoea: *ajirno* (caused by indigestion and food poisoning, and which accounts for about 50 per cent of cases); *arnasha* (contains mucus, cause unknown, and which accounts for 33 per cent of cases); *dud haga* (caused by ingesting 'polluted' breast milk, and which accounts for 12 per cent of cases); and a severe, watery dehydrating form, accounting for 5 per cent of cases (Chowdhury et al., 1988). These local sub-categories are not found in the current global classification system.

A further change may take place with the recognition of a disease as abnormal. This includes a range of conditions where medicine has changed its view on a condition. For example, in the nineteenth century ptosis was based on the erroneous belief that the large bowel should not be free to move within the abdomen, leading to operations to attach the bowel to the abdominal wall; or night starvation in the 1930s, which was based on the belief that people suffer from low sugar levels as they sleep, and should therefore take a sugary drink before going to bed. These practices are no longer promoted.

Finally, a change may take place due to the uncovering of previously rare conditions. This can happen when there is a reduction or elimination of other prevalent conditions, bringing to prominence a previously unnoticed condition. This is explained in the following extract from an editorial in the *Lancet* in 1993, entitled the 'Rise and fall of diseases':

The apparent newness of diseases has fuelled fierce debates. Many major scourges of our 20th century industrialised world received their proper names only in the second half of the last century or early in this one; examples include coronary heart disease, schizophrenia, and rheumatoid arthritis. Many doctors cannot credit that diseases which to us stand so clearly on their own might have escaped the recognition of medical professionals of bygone times – hence the idea that these are diseases 'caused' by civilisation. Medawar proposed an alternative view – that most diseases that afflict us from middle age onwards might simply represent 'unfavourable' genes that have accumulated to express themselves in the second half of our lives. This could never be corrected by any evolutionary pressure since such pressures act only on the first half of our lives: once we have reproduced it does not greatly matter that we grow 'sans teeth, sans eyes, sans taste, sans everything'. Sexual attraction and physical vigour have served their turn and thereafter all types of haphazardly accumulated decay can freely express themselves. Civilisation, which has wiped out famine and pestilence in industrialised society, is therefore not the cause of our chronic diseases; it merely unveiled what our genes had lurking in store for us for centuries, if not millennia, as we now live long enough to see these genes massively expressing themselves. Such large-scale expression has greatly facilitated the 'discovery' of the diseases of civilisation – i.e., their description as separate entities. This notion finds support in the writings of historical demographers and historians who believe that our 'western' chronic disease pattern already existed among the few well-to-do people of the past, who were slightly better nourished, slightly more exempt from pestilences, and lived somewhat longer. If true, lifestyle changes will be of little avail.

Reprinted from *Lancet* (1993) Rise and fall of diseases, *Lancet*, 341 (8838): 151–2, with permission from Elsevier.

The importance of disease classification

You may be wondering whether it matters greatly how diseases are categorized and if the categories change over time. But as you will explore in this section, the way that diseases are classified has important social as well as economic implications, and can even influence the type of society you live in.

In his paper entitled 'In search of non-disease', Richard Smith (2002) outlines some of these important implications. He highlights both the benefits as well as some drawbacks for individuals of the labelling of a disease. Some examples are outlined below:

- *Eligibility for treatment*: if something is deemed to be a disease, then the person is eligible for treatment. A contemporary example of such a condition is myalgic encephalomyelisitis. Before 2002 the condition was not identified as a disease, and sufferers had difficulty seeking recognition for their condition, and thus treatment. However, even though the condition is now recognized, there is still some uncertainty about whether effective treatment is available.
- *Employment rights*: if a condition is recognized as a disease, then it can have important implications for employment rights. Repetitive strain injury is an example of a condition that has now been recognized as a disease. This has implications for the way that employers need to protect staff from the condition, and support them in the event that they are affected.
- *Insurance compensation*: the categorization of a condition as a disease can also affect whether the sufferer is eligible for compensation. A common example of this in the UK is the diagnosis of 'whiplash' in car drivers and passengers, resulting from a collision.

- *Social security rights*: if a condition is categorized as a disease, then there may be implications for social security rights. An example of this is the case of drug abuse. When categorized as a disease, for which there is treatment, accepting this treatment has been used as a 'conditionality' for receipt of social security benefits.

How diseases are classified also has implication for the way that the aetiology of disease is understood, and how diseases are recorded on death certificates. Recent data suggest that only one in four death certificates accurately reflect how a person died. This means that not only might families be misinformed on the nature of their relative's death, but that research based on death certificate data may not be accurate. This has important implications for the types of policies developed to address causes of death in the population, and ultimately how resources for health are allocated.

Finally, the idea of labelling a condition as a disease has led some commentators to warn against the 'medicalization' of normal physiological processes. You will look at this issue in more detail below.

Medicalization

The term 'medicalization' is not a new term but has received increased attention in recent years. Essentially, it is concerned with 'defining a problem in medical terms, usually as an illness or disorder, or using medical intervention to treat it' (Conrad, 2005, cited in Bell and Figert, 2012).

As you have already seen, it is not always obvious what is a disease and what is not. Several commentators point to an increasing trend to view a number of common issues, previously regarded as a normal part of everyday life, in medical terms, and treat them with a medical intervention. These problems include such diverse issues as baldness (Moynihan et al., 2002), erectile dysfunction (Moynihan et al., 2002), and childbirth (Shaw, 2013). Some commentators have also pointed to the medicalization of non-communicable or chronic diseases, such as obesity-related chronic disease (Thorpe and Philyaw, 2012). Moynihan et al. (2002) have outlined a number of potentially negative consequences of the trend, including:

- reinforcing stereotypes
- financial waste
- iatrogenic illness
- diversion of attention from political or other social issues.

In some cases, the role of the corporate sector has been questioned, being seen to promote the medicalization of issues for marketing purposes, a process that has been termed 'disease mongering' (Moynihan et al., 2002).

As you have noted from the preceding discussion, labelling a condition as a disease can have social and economic implications for the individual as well as society.

Activity 3.2

Take a few moments to think of conditions that you think are being medicalized in a country with which you are familiar. Do you think that this trend will lead to better health? Do you see any drawbacks?

Feedback

You may have thought of some of the conditions mentioned above, such as baldness or childbirth or a non-communicable disease. You may have listed drawbacks such as an increasing focus on issues that need to be 'treated' and the cost that this will involve, either for individuals or health care systems. You may also have noted that a focus on pharmaceutical intervention has resulted in less emphasis on other potential strategies, which may have wider benefits beyond the issue in question, and for long-term health in the population, such as increased exercise (Moynihan et al., 2002). Alternatively, you may have cited some positive examples, such as eligibility for treatment that may benefit some individuals.

Culture and disease

As you have seen, the perception of disease has a cultural dimension, affecting both self-assessment and professional judgement. There is a large body of literature from medical anthropology describing the cultural context of disease. Many of the underlying differences in health services that are seen between countries are based on cultural factors.

What is culture?

Culture is a set of values, beliefs, and attitudes that are associated with a social system. For example, when comparing traditional Indian (Ayurvedic) medicine to western medicine, you may analyse the *material culture* and compare the medical tools and products used by both systems. You can also analyse the *non-material culture* and examine the ideas underlying Ayurvedic and western medicine. These ideas are the different *beliefs*, *values*, and *norms* that are reflected in the medical theory and practice of both systems. You may, for example, compare the methods of generating medical knowledge and classifying diseases. Or, you may compare the beliefs and norms underlying the self-perception of disease in the two cultures.

In her book, *Medicine and Culture* published in 1988, Lynn Payer explored these differences from the perspective of a medical journalist who has studied health care in the USA and Europe. Her original interest in the subject of medical differences was stimulated by her own experiences of receiving care in different countries for fibroids, a common benign condition of the uterus. This was diagnosed when living in France where doctors recommended a limited operation that simply removed the fibroid and preserved the uterus and thus her ability to have children. In contrast, in the USA, doctors recommended a hysterectomy (removal of the uterus) as this would remove any chance of subsequently developing cancer of the cervix or uterus. Her interpretation of this was that 'therapeutic recommendations were influenced less by the facts of my case than by how much the culture in which they operated valued the ability to have children'.

This led her to look at other international differences in professional judgements. She discovered that:

> *'Some of the most commonly prescribed drugs in France, drugs to dilate the cerebral blood vessels, are considered ineffective in England and America; an obligatory immunization against tuberculosis in France, BCG is almost impossible to obtain in the United States. German doctors prescribe from six to seven times the amount of digitalis-like [heart] drugs as their colleagues in France and England, but they prescribe fewer antibiotics, with some German doctors maintaining antibiotics shouldn't be used unless the patient is sick enough to be in the hospital. Doses of the same drug may vary drastically, with some nationalities getting ten to twenty times what other nationals get. French people have seven times the chance of getting drugs in suppository form as do Americans.'*

This helped explain the differences in surgical rates between countries that were being revealed in the 1970s. Rates in the USA were about twice those of England, a difference that has persisted to today. Some differences were even more marked: mastectomies (breast removal) were three times higher in New England than in England even though the rate of breast cancer was similar; appendectomies were three times higher in Germany than other high-income countries.

Payer also noticed that

> *'the same clinical signs may even receive different diagnoses. Often, all one must do to acquire a disease is to enter a country where that disease is recognized – leaving the country will either cure the malady or turn it into something else. The American schizophrenic of a few years ago might well have found his disease called manic-depressive disease or even neurosis had he sought a second opinion in Britain; in France he likely would have been diagnosed as having a delusional psychosis.'*

The effect of cultural differences can even be seen in variations in attribution of cause of death.

Marked differences in professional views between countries have three practical implications. First, there is a danger of drawing unjustified conclusions from international comparisons. This can also be seen in historic changes in medical culture. In the UK, some of the increased incidence of ischaemic heart disease is due to a change from the previous use of the term 'degenerative heart disease' for such patients. This inevitably inflates the perceived size of the 'epidemic' of ischaemic heart disease, increasing the scale of research funding and provision of cardiac services at the expense of other areas of clinical need and the public's perception of risk of heart disease.

The second implication is the opportunity that cultural differences provide for increasing our understanding of disease and health care. Payer identified an example of the use of such natural experiments: 'French doctors have widely prescribed calcium for a number of years, and a closer examination of osteoporosis rates there might help illuminate the role of calcium in this disease.'

She also identified a third implication:

'Many of the medical mistakes made in each country can be best understood by cultural biases that blind both the medical profession and patients, causing them to accept some treatments too quickly and other treatments reluctantly or not at all. Understanding the cultural basis for these mistakes can perhaps prevent them – or at least lessen their impact.'

Activity 3.3

Cultural differences have implications for health services research and for managing health systems. Suggest why awareness of international variations due to cultural differences is important.

Feedback

Two of the consequences you may have suggested are:

1 If international variations in patterns of disease partly reflect cultural differences, accepting the differences as being real may result in misleading views as to the causes of disease.
2 International variations can be used to compare the effectiveness and efficiency of different services as they provide a 'natural experiment'.

✎   **Activity 3.4**

Compare the drug consumption for different categories of disease between the UK and Germany as shown in Table 3.1. Does it reflect the cultural differences between the two countries mentioned by Payer? Make brief notes on your comparison.

Table 3.1 Pharmaceutical consumption in the UK and Germany: defined daily doses in 1990

Indication	Germany	UK
Cardiovascular system	607	234
Respiratory system	583	435
Digestive system	511	406
Central nervous system	323	441
Systematic hormone replacement	28	59

Source: Data from Fink-Anthe (1992).

Feedback

Alhough there are several important factors determining prescribing behaviour, such as guidelines, incentives, and marketing efforts of the drug industry, some differences can only be explained by cultural reasons. The largest differences above relate to treatment of diseases of the cardiovascular and the central nervous system. The observed high level of cardiovascular drugs in Germany is consistent with Payer's view. The high levels of tranquillizers and antidepressants prescribed in the UK have been attributed to the cultural attitude of 'keeping a stiff upper lip' in times of personal troubles.

You may think that we now have all the answers to the questions of disease and that it was only in the past that mistakes in classification occurred. Like our predecessors, however, we are only as wise as our available knowledge. In addition, as you have seen, scientific knowledge is only one aspect that is determining our classification of disease.

Summary

The concept of disease is dependent on social and cultural factors. Medical knowledge is based on categorizing states of ill health into discrete diseases. Analysing why these categories change over time provides insight into how medical knowledge is generated. In this chapter, you have learned about the cultural beliefs, values, and norms underlying medical thinking. Cultural factors account for many of the differences observed in international comparisons of health services. The current trend to medicalize many everyday problems is a contemporary example of how social and cultural factors help shape our ideas about disease.

In this chapter, you have seen that our ideas about disease change over time. Care must be taken, therefore, so as not to overestimate the confidence that is placed in current classifications. In the next chapter, you will look at what influences the prevailing set of beliefs, or medical paradigm, and how this impacts on the view of disease.

References

Bell, S.E. and Figert, A.E. (2012) Medicalization and pharmaceuticalization at the intersections: looking backward, sideways and forward, *Social Science and Medicine*, 75 (5): 775–83.

Black, N.A. (1984) Is glue ear a modern phenomenon? A historical review of the medical literature, *Clinical Otolaryngology*, 9 (3): 155–63.

Chowdhury, M., Vaughan, P.V. and Abed, F.H. (1988) Use and safety of home-made oral rehydration solutions: an epidemiological evaluation from Bangladesh, *International Journal of Epidemiology*, 17 (3): 655–65.

Conrad, P. (2005) The shifting engines of medicalization, *Journal of Health and Social Behavior*, 46 (1): 3–14.

Fink-Anthe, C. (1992) Kulturell beeinflußte Therapiegewohnheiten: Bedeutung für den europäischen Markt, *Deutsche Apotheker Zeitung*, 29: 1534–9.

King, L. (1954) What is disease?, *Philosophy of Science*, 21 (3): 193–203.

Lancet (1993) Rise and fall of diseases, *Lancet*, 341 (8838): 151–2.

Moynihan, R., Heath, I. and Henry, D. (2002) Selling sickness: the pharmaceutical industry and disease mongering, *British Medical Journal*, 324 (7342): 886–91.

Payer, L. (1988) *Medicine and Culture*. New York: Henry Holt.

Shaw, J.C. (2013) The medicalization of birth and midwifery as resistance, *Health Care for Women International*, 34 (6): 522–36.

Smith, R. (2002) In search of 'non-disease', *British Medical Journal*, 324 (7342): 883–5.

Stehbens, W.E. (1987) An appraisal of the epidemic rise of coronary heart disease and its decline, *Lancet*, 1 (8533): 606–11.

Thorpe, K.E. and Philyaw, M. (2012) The medicalization of chronic disease and costs, *Annual Review of Public Health*, 33: 409–23.

4 Medical paradigms

Overview

In the previous chapter, you learnt how medical knowledge is generated. In this chapter, you will explore the concept of medical paradigms. You will learn how the concepts of illness have changed over time and what this has meant for the health services provided, including recent developments in precision medicine. You will examine the implications of these shifts for the roles of health care professionals and patients. You will also look more closely at the role of clinicians in the development of medical knowledge.

Learning objectives

After working through this chapter, you will be able to:

- outline the concept of medical paradigms
- distinguish the major shifts in medical paradigms that have occurred in western medicine
- understand the implications of different medical paradigms for health service provision and the roles of health professionals and patients
- discuss the contributions that clinicians make to the development of medical knowledge and the limitations of this

Key terms

Case series: Study of a series of cases to identify common or recurring features.

Case study: Observation and analysis of a single case to generate a hypothesis.

Discourse: The way language is used in a particular area.

Holism: The conceptualization of a system as a whole and the belief that the whole is greater than the sum of its parts.

> **Medical cosmology:** The study of medical paradigms.
>
> **Medical paradigm:** The prevailing thoughts and knowledge about health and disease.
>
> **Precision medicine:** The application of specific knowledge of individual variability in the choice of prevention and treatment strategies.
>
> **Reductionism:** Consideration of the component parts rather than the whole organism or organization.
>
> **Surveillance medicine:** The widespread monitoring of the population for symptoms of disease or for established conditions.

Medical paradigms

As you learnt in the previous chapter, categories of diseases can change. Disease classification, however, is just one aspect of medical knowledge. Other aspects include:

- Aetiology (the cause of disease)
- Pathogenesis (the way disease develops)
- Pathology (the underlying fault or abnormality in a tissue or organ)
- Natural history of disease (the way a disease develops and progresses)
- Treatment.

The categories of disease thus sit within a wider medical paradigm that reflects the prevailing thoughts and knowledge at any given time. These thoughts and knowledge need to be internally consistent if they are to represent a coherent set of views on all aspects of medicine. A range of factors such as the research methods in use, the teaching approaches, the way health care practitioners perceive their patients, as well as what patients expect from practitioners, are all part of, and will all inform, the prevailing paradigm.

The study of medical paradigms, known as 'medical cosmology', can help you understand important aspects of health care. You will explore the changing nature of medical paradigms in more detail in the next sections.

The importance of language

In the first instance, it is important to be aware that the views held on a subject are related to the use of language. Indeed, one field of research in medical paradigms focuses on examining written and spoken material to discover the underlying thoughts on a subject. For example, as you learnt in Section 1, the views, as well as the language used to describe mental illness, have changed significantly over the last two hundred years.

The French philosopher Michel Foucault (1926–1984) highlighted the importance of language for structuring knowledge and exerting power. To him, the way language (writing, talking) is used directs people to understand issues in certain ways that constitute their perception and knowledge of the world. He examined the development of language in certain areas of social life and how this process was used to exert power. He called the way language is used in a particular area *discourse*. Powerful groups can influence discourses in a particular area and, vice versa, a particular discourse creates power by limiting the meaning of language.

In one of his key books, *Madness and Civilization* (1967), Foucault explored the use of language, like an archaeologist digging through layer after layer to trace how, in the western world, madness – which was once thought to be divinely inspired – came to be thought of as mental illness. He showed that, depending on the historical period, the mentally ill were initially treated as outcasts, then later were imprisoned and treated as criminals, before reforms in the nineteenth century gave way to humanitarian treatment in asylums, and the rise of psychiatry as a profession.

Since then, the discourse on mental illness has been dominated by psychiatry. But is it changing again? With the advent of effective drugs, much mental illness can be treated in the community. With decarceration from the large asylums that were a feature of nineteenth- and early twentieth-century care, professions other than psychiatry are gaining influence on the discourse. As a result, the way in which people with such conditions are viewed has been gradually changing from 'inmates' to 'patients' and, more recently, to 'clients'.

Why study changing discourse and shifts in the medical paradigm?

You may be asking, what benefits are to be gained from studying the changing discourse on medicine and the medical paradigm? As you saw above, understanding the way a disease is viewed can have implications for those who are ill. A study of medical paradigms is therefore needed for three main reasons:

1 It will help you understand the views held on patients and diseases.
2 It will provide you with insights into some of the universal problems of modern health care, and the interaction between practitioners and patients.
3 It will help you understand the strengths and limitations of clinical research.

You will now look at the major medical paradigms in western medical knowledge. Jewson (1976) identified three major shifts relating to pre-nineteenth-century, nineteenth-century, and twentieth-century medicine, respectively. Having explored these you will look at what is happening in the twenty-first century.

Pre-nineteenth-century bedside medicine

Before the nineteenth century, doctors' knowledge and observation of patients were largely confined to their visits to their middle- and upper-class patients (who were their patrons), in their own homes. At this time, the prevailing explanation of death and disease was the imbalance in the four humours (key fluids) of the body, which were designated – blood, choler (yellow bile), phlegm, and black bile. This was a holistic view of medicine in which illness was seen as a psychosomatic disturbance of the whole person. The basis of the doctor's understanding was speculation and inference. Their role was to predict the future (prognosis) and to apply the relevant therapy, such as bleeding the patient. The close relationship between the doctor and their patron meant that an individual doctor's theory and practice were greatly influenced by their patron's views.

Nineteenth-century hospital medicine

By the nineteenth century, there was growing urbanization in Europe and North America as large numbers in these populations moved to the cities in search of jobs and higher incomes, leaving behind their rural lives. One outcome of this was the development of institutions to look after those who were not benefiting from the new opportunities (i.e. the sick, the elderly, and those with a disability). These institutions had the effect of bringing together large numbers of sick persons in one place, and the employment of doctors to provide them with basic care. This presented the opportunity for doctors to study groups of sick persons under their care and to observe associations and trends. In addition, when patients died, doctors were able to undertake post-mortems (autopsies) to see what had been going on in the body (pathology). At the same time, there were advances in physical sciences. The application of new understanding in chemistry and physics led to the development of tools for doctors to investigate the body, including the stethoscope to listen to the chest, the otoscope to examine ears, and the ophthalmoscope to look into the eyes. The combination of these developments meant that doctors started to employ statistically orientated clinical observation rather than speculation and inference. Illnesses were seen as organic lesions and patients were 'cases' of specific diseases, as the classification of diseases developed. The role of the doctor shifted from prognosis to diagnosis and the control of medical knowledge also shifted to the doctors and those leading the profession.

Twentieth-century laboratory medicine

The technological developments of the twentieth century allowed for the increasing investigation of organs, tissues, and cells within the body, through invasive and more recently less invasive techniques. Patients were seen as a complex of cells to be understood. Illness was seen as a biological process, and diagnosis shifted from the ward to the laboratory. Control of medical knowledge also shifted again, this time to the laboratory scientist. The doctor's role was focused on the analysis of the information received from the laboratory and the explanation of what was wrong. This focus on distinct, single processes has been called a *reductionist* view, and is in contrast to the earlier *holistic* view that tries to conceptualize and understand the whole of the complex system.

However, there was also a reappearance of a more holistic approach in the twentieth century, seeing illness in terms of constitutional disorders such as endocrine dysfunction and allergies. In addition, there was greater recognition of the social and behavioural factors underlying disease. There was a rise in 'surveillance medicine' (Armstrong, 1995) with the monitoring of the health of the population on a large scale through regular screening sessions. Armstrong (1995) highlights how surveillance medicine encompasses those who are healthy, as well as those who are sick, with the inclusion of risk factors as markers of potential illness, going beyond the previous reliance on signs and symptoms of disease, and requiring a 'problematization of normal'. Compare this with the concept of 'medicalization' discussed in the previous chapter. The shift to monitoring health in the population was also associated with a transfer in the control of medical knowledge once again, this time to the epidemiologists who were responsible for the mapping of risk (Nettleton, 2004).

Twenty-first-century precision medicine

The early twenty-first century has seen the rise of what has been termed 'precision medicine', an approach that uses 'prevention and treatment strategies that take individual variability into account' (Collins and Varmus, 2015). While the idea of personalizing medicine has been around for some time, precision medicine has come into its own in recent years with the genetic revolution and the development of technology that enables the identification of the specific gene patterns that are associated with disease. Over the last decade, the costs of the necessary technology to undertake human genome sequencing have reduced dramatically, making access to such techniques more widespread.

These advances have led to increased options for tailored treatment. For example, it is now possible to identify the specific genetic make-up of a cancer and to apply the treatment known to act on this make-up. It is also possible to say with some certainty whether a person will benefit from a particular treatment or not, with implications for who is treated.

Whether this will be a new paradigm is yet to be seen, but it is certainly viewed by governments as an important area of investment. In the USA, President Obama launched a new research initiative to promote the role of precision medicine as part of his 2015 State of the Union address, while the UK government has launched a centre for precision medicine (*The Precision Medicine Catapult*). Both initiatives seek to promote new ways to treat disease as well as build a knowledge base in this area (Collins and Varmus, 2015).

At the same time, commentators note that current systems will need to be updated to ensure that precision medicine delivers on its anticipated benefits. This includes updating systems to handle a different type of data; modifying disease classifications to take account of the new knowledge; training doctors and other health staff working with patients so that they are able to explain the options available; and the involvement of the public themselves in decision-making on the future of precision medicine (Mirnezami et al., 2012).

A further development in the twenty-first century associated with the rise of technology is the notion of 'E-scaped' medicine, where knowledge is no longer the purview of a particular professional group (whether doctor or scientist) but is located, as a result of technology, in a space that is accessible by all. In this case, evidence from a variety of sources may sit side by side, to be utilized by both the patient and the professional (Nettleton, 2004).

✎ Activity 4.1

The changing medical paradigms have influenced the nature of holism. The loss of the holistic view in the early twentieth century may explain the demand for alternative therapies. In the previous chapter, you explored attitudes towards traditional healers. Now think of the *approach* they use and contrast it to western medicine. Are there, besides the paradigm of western medicine, any other medical paradigms in your country, which may have preserved the holistic approach to illness? Make brief notes as to any contrasting approaches you may have thought of.

Feedback

Many of the traditional medical systems appear to be based on a holistic approach, as are animist healers and the traditional medicine in India or China. Despite the many unproven therapies, these systems have maintained their attractiveness to patients. For example, the Indian government supports traditional medicine and it has been argued that traditional medical practitioners are closer to people's own perception of health than is western medicine (Ramesh and Hyma, 1981). You may also have identified schools of thought that evolved in response to modern medicine, including anthroposophic medicine and psychosomatic medicine – these have refocused on illness as a process affecting the whole person.

Dangers of the biomedical/clinical paradigm

As a manager or as a researcher you need to rely on current disease classification, despite the fact that medical knowledge is conditional. You also need to be aware that acceptance of established knowledge has a danger of restricting and limiting useful new ideas and it can be extremely difficult to challenge established views.

✎ Activity 4.2

This activity invites you to explore the potential dangers of depending on hospital clinicians' knowledge of disease. Write brief notes on what those dangers might be, and then compare your notes with the feedback below.

Feedback

Some of the inherent dangers are:

1 Hospital clinicians only observe the diseased, so they may be unaware of the existence of people with similar symptoms who are not seeking care. For example, most people with chest pain seen by a cardiologist will have heart disease, yet a general practitioner may see many others with chest pain and not refer them because the pain originates from other causes.
2 Observations are confined to the clinical setting. The environment itself might induce ill health. For example, some people will have a raised blood pressure in hospital because they find the setting stressful, so-called 'white-coat' hypertension.
3 Clinicians are unable to assess factors outside the individual that may be contributing to a patient's ill health, such as their job or their housing.
4 Clinicians inadvertently teach their patients to adhere to established categories of disease. The dangers of complicity between clinicians and patients has long been recognized:

> ... theories tell clinicians what to look for, what to ignore, and to act upon. Of course, they also tell patients what to see, for patients are schooled both directly and indirectly in the realities of illness and of medical disorders. As a result, given different background assumptions, different things will stand out in the patient's experience of his or her illness. In short, prevailing biomedical viewpoints fashion the life-world of patients so that their disorders appear already shaped in part by the scientific understandings of disease. (Engelhardt, 1981)

5 Clinicians may be reluctant to challenge established views. This was succinctly described by Richard Asher (1972), a British doctor, in a warning to young trainee doctors:

> We refrain from speaking about things that we observe when they are not listed in the official phenomena of the text-book description; apart from that we refrain from speaking our own opinions when they conflict too violently with generally accepted thought, or when they are greatly at variance with the opinions of those we fear. It is probably to our advantage that we do so, but it is of no advantage to the forward march of medical science.

Given these limitations, the contribution of clinicians to understanding health and disease is inevitably limited. However, that does not mean it is unimportant. It is a key source of hypotheses (or new ideas). Generally, clinical research takes two forms:

- the *case study* – detection of the odd, unusual or rare observation;
- the *case series* – identification of common, recurring associations.

The skills required for detecting associations in a series of cases are much greater than those required for identifying single, odd events. It has been likened to the difference between noticing a very rare bird in your garden (case study) and noticing twice as many of a common bird that is a frequent visitor to your garden (case series). Most of us would manage the former but only the more observant would spot the latter.

Summary

The concept of a medical paradigm takes account of all aspects (the discourse) of medicine at a given time. You have seen how shifts have taken place over several centuries in the western medical paradigm: from bedside medicine to hospital medicine and from there to laboratory medicine, and most recently the importance of 'surveillance medicine' and 'E-scaped' medicine. Along with these shifts, the changing conceptualization of illness from a psychosomatic disturbance to a biochemical process to the mapping of risk, has changed the relationship between sick individuals – and even healthy individuals – and health care practitioners. Western medicine has also shifted from a holistic to a reductionist perspective. The reappearance of the holistic approach and an increased awareness of the social and behavioural views of illness are important aspects of the current debate on health services. The recent rise of precision medicine has opened up the options for more targeted treatment of diseases, though whether this is a new paradigm is not yet certain. However, it will likely spearhead changes in the way that medicine is delivered. Finally, this chapter considered the strengths and limitations of the methods that clinicians use in formulating medical knowledge. As a manager or a researcher, there is a need to question basic assumptions about any diseased state and disease categorization before considering detailed analyses or policy decisions. You should always first ask whether you can accept the implicit assumptions that are being made.

References

Armstrong, D. (1995) The rise of surveillance medicine, *Sociology of Health and Illness*, 17 (3): 393–404.

Asher, R. (1972) *Talking Sense*. London: Pitman Medical.

Collins, F.S. and Varmus, H. (2015) A new initiative on precision medicine, *New England Journal of Medicine*, 372 (9): 793–5.

Engelhardt, H.T. (1981) Clinical judgement, *Metamedicine*, 2: 301–17.

Foucault, M. (1967) *Madness and Civilization: A history of insanity in the age of reason* (trans. R. Howard). London: Tavistock.

Jewson, N. (1976) The disappearance of the sick man from the medical cosmology 1770–1870, *Sociology*, 10 (2): 225–44.

Mirnezami, R., Nicholson, J. and Darzi, A. (2012) Preparing for precision medicine, *New England Journal of Medicine*, 366 (6): 489–91.

Nettleton, S. (2004) The emergence of escaped medicine, *Sociology*, 38 (4): 661–80.

Ramesh, A. and Hyma, B. (1981) Traditional Indian medicine in practice in an Indian metropolitan city, *Social Science and Medicine*, 15 (1): 69–81.

Health care professionals

5

Overview

In this chapter, you will examine another key input into health services, namely that of health staff. Building on the earlier discussion on the role of formal and lay care in Chapter 2, this chapter explores what is meant by a professional health care worker, why some health care providers have a particular status, and what this means for health services. You will compare the professional development of different health staff, and how practitioners from different medical systems co-exist. You will be introduced to different sociological views on professional autonomy. Finally, you will explore a number of contemporary challenges to health care professions, and how the medical profession is changing, including the growth of hybrid professionals. You will also look at the implications of globalization for the availability of health care professionals.

Learning objectives

After working through this chapter, you will be able to:

- identify what is meant by a profession and how it differs from an occupation
- identify factors contributing to the power of professions
- compare and contrast medicine and nursing as professions
- understand some of the contemporary challenges to health care professionals
- understand the role of hybrid professionals
- understand the implications of globalization for health care professionals

Key terms

Ambulatory care: Health care provided to patients without admitting them to hospital such as general practice, out-patient clinics, and day care.

Global workforce crisis: A shortage of health workers across the world that has been exacerbated by the global demand for health care.

Hybrid professionals: A professional embodying the working practices and principles of two different roles in their work.

Ideal type: A hypothetical model of a complex real phenomenon that emphasizes its most salient features.

Ideology: A set of beliefs, values, and attitudes used to justify and legitimize power.

Power: The ability to influence – and in particular to control – others, events, and resources.

Profession: An occupation based on specified knowledge and training and regulated standards of performance.

Professionalization: A process whereby an occupation achieves the more independent status of a profession.

Reprofessionalization: A change in the nature of how the (medical) profession is viewed.

Why study professions?

You saw in Chapter 4 how medicine has gained its status through the ability to determine the discourse on illness. But how have the main actors, the doctors, achieved their leading status in health care? And why is it important to study the professional development of health care occupations?

As you will explore in this chapter, the concept of 'profession' is central to our understanding of the relationship between the different actors within health services. It also provides insight into the relationship between health workers and the public. Understanding these relationships is essential for the good management of services. For example, managers need to be aware of the influence of professional groups and organizations and to be able to anticipate where there may be resistance to change.

What is a professional?

In common language use, any occupation may be referred to as a profession. However, in a stricter sense there are some important characteristics assigned to professions that distinguish them from occupations in general.

A 'profession' may be distinguished by its claim to most or all of the following characteristics:

- A body of specialized knowledge and skills that is built on rigorous and lengthy academic training.
- A (legal) monopoly over practice that regulates entry into the profession and specifies the requirements for training and qualifications to practice.
- A code of ethics/practice that provides the rules within which the members of the profession operate. This is generally self-policed, thus providing autonomy of practice.
- A degree of altruism that incorporates a service ideology or vocation.

These factors are based on the concept of an 'ideal type' as proposed by the German sociologist, Max Weber, in 1947. Note that 'ideal' here is not meant in the sense of desirable (or normative) but in the sense of a pure, abstract construct (i.e. an idea).

A combination of these factors will determine the position, as well as the financial rewards, that are afforded to a particular profession. This results in the privileged position given to some professions in society.

You can use the 'ideal type' characteristics to contrast the professional status of different occupations, or to compare the process of professionalization in different countries.

✎ Activity 5.1

Choose a country with which you are familiar. Using the ideal type characteristics outlined above, identify and list examples of occupations that have achieved professional status in the country you have chosen.

Feedback

You are likely to have listed law and medicine in the first instance, followed perhaps by occupations such as dentistry, architecture, accountancy, teaching, and nursing. The extent of the professionalization of these latter professions varies between countries. The first established professionals were self-employed and charged fees. Members of these professions were granted a privileged status through government regulation. In most countries, professionalization is an ongoing process, with a number of occupations trying to professionalize themselves by forming associations and striving to establish recognition for ethical standards, formalized training, and specialized knowledge. A few have achieved professional status, but probably none has achieved a professional status as complete as that accorded to law or medicine.

Two key factors determine the dominance that a certain profession is able to exert within society. These are (1) its relation to markets and (2) its relation to other occupations (Allsop and Saks, 2002). The status relative to other occupations can be assessed by:

- *Wealth*: higher income, as a result of a better position in the marketplace.
- *Prestige*: the esteem in which others hold the group.
- *Power*: the ability to influence decisions and other occupations in the field.

From a sociological and political perspective, power is a key concept in understanding the behaviour of social systems. In Chapter 4, you learnt about the relationship between language and power. Power can be conceptualized as the ability to influence – or in Weber's definition, to control – others, events, and resources. In this view, power can be *coercive* by using force, or it can be based on *authority*, which is accepted by others and seen as legitimate. There are also more subtle forms of power, such as the power of *non-decision-making* and, as you have seen earlier, the power to shape the beliefs and values of others.

The power of the medical profession

The medical profession enjoys a particular position of trust within the population as well as a position of power. Historically, the position of power has developed as a result of the profession achieving a legal and ideological monopoly. Factors facilitating this process include the scientific background of medical knowledge underpinning the profession, and the reliance on organized education.

It is possible to identify three processes by which the medical profession has realized a dominant position in health care (Freidson, 1988):

1 *Subjugation*: the medical profession has ensured a position of power over other staff undertaking similar roles (e.g. nursing).
2 *Limitation*: the medical profession has successfully excluded others undertaking similarly skilled roles (e.g. dentistry).
3 *Exclusion*: the medical profession has outlined what will, and thus will not, be included in the concept of medicine (e.g. herbalists in UK).

It is also possible to see the role of monopoly as well as markets at play in the positioning of medicine in the examples of the UK and US contexts. In the UK, the Medical Act of 1858 joined together the three main groups of medical practitioners at the time – the Royal College of Physicians, the Surgeons, and the General Practitioners (Apothecaries) – into one register, and thus established the General Medical Council. Since this point, the Council has had the role of overseeing and regulating the range of doctors engaged in health care and ensuring good medical practice. Note that it excludes dentists despite their role as dental surgeons. A similar body, the American Medical Association, controls all admissions to medical schools and licences to practise in the USA.

The following activity will give you the opportunity to reflect on the relative power of doctors in health services.

✎ Activity 5.2

The following terms represent key aspects of professional power. Suggest an example of each as it relates to doctors:

- Technical expertise
- Authority
- Clientele
- Uncertainty
- Relationship to other professions.

Feedback

Compare your explanations with those in Table 5.1. Are they broadly in line?

Table 5.1 Key aspects of professional power

Professional power is based on:	Example relating to doctors
Technical expertise	Scientific background of medical knowledge, special skills, e.g. surgical operations
Authority	Doctors provide a widely acknowledged view on health and illness; they are accepted as persons to give ultimate advice in health matters
Clientele	Unlike many other occupations, doctors have individual clients (patients), who engage in a personal relationship based on trust
Uncertainty	The uncertainty of need for health care and of the outcomes of care leads people to seek professional advice from experts
Relationship with other professionals	Medicine has developed as the lead profession in health services. For example, doctors are better paid and occupy higher ranks in the hierarchy than other health workers

Comparing the professions of medicine and nursing

You have seen how medicine has developed as a profession. However, nursing is also a profession. The relationship between nursing and medicine is an interesting example of the importance of gender in power differentials. You have already noted that the profession of nursing has been historically subjugated to medicine. In addition, nursing has traditionally been dominated by women, while medicine has been dominated by men. This is changing and the number of women entering medicine is growing, while men are increasingly entering the nursing profession. However, gender perceptions within both professions are slow to change. There is evidence that men are subject to discrimination in their education and work as nurses, and can feel isolated by the female gender bias in the profession (Kouta and Kaite, 2011; McLaughlin et al., 2010). In medicine, the speciality of surgery is still dominated by men, while women make up the majority of general practitioners (GPs).

Phil Strong, a sociologist, and Jane Robinson, a nurse, provided valuable insights into the power relations between different groups of health workers in their classic study on doctors and nurses in the UK in the late 1980s (Strong and Robinson, 1990).

The authors identified a number of reasons for the more limited professional development of nurses compared with doctors. These differences were associated with:

- lack of independence – nurses are more bound into hierarchy and quasi-military discipline;
- lack of autonomy in clinical judgement;
- lack of own scientific knowledge and language;
- lack of solidarity and syndicalist mode (i.e. through a union) of interest representation;
- lack of influence on decision-making.

It is important to note that many of these problems are related to the traditional gender role of women in society at this time, with nursing often being viewed as women's work and seen as a domestic service that does not require expert knowledge.

Internationally, the status of nursing varies, as do the requirements for training, career prospects, and payment levels, relative to doctors across different countries. Different curricula and job entry requirements may also exist within a country between ambulatory care and hospitals. The nurse/doctor ratio may also vary widely, again a reflection to some extent of the professional status of nurses. Strengthening nursing education and professional development is high on the agenda of many countries. Where independent nurse practitioners have been introduced, this has often been seen as a challenge to the medical profession.

Activity 5.3

Think about the professional status of nurses in a country with which you are familiar. What key factors are influencing their professional status in this country?

Feedback

Depending on the country you have chosen, you may have listed a number of factors – both historical and current – that have impacted on the status of nurses. You may have chosen a country where many of the decisions about health staff are made by policy-makers with a medical, rather than nursing, background, and there may be a reluctance to concede roles to nurses that have historically been undertaken by doctors, even though these roles are already being performed by nurses in other contexts. The entry requirements for nursing may also influence the status of nurses in your chosen context. Or, you may have identified a gender perspective in terms of status. For example, you may have chosen a country in which increasing numbers of men are entering the nursing profession, and this may be having a positive effect on the status of nursing in this context.

The role of managers in health care

An important challenge to the role of both medical and nursing professions is the rise of management cadres. The function of management is to ensure strategic decision-making and the pursuit of goals that are in the best interests of an organization. The question is who is best placed to perform these functions in health care? In particular, does the professional authority afforded to the medical profession help or hinder the management of services?

One view of the relationship between managers and other health care staff is what Strauss (1963, 1964, cited in Allen, 1997) called a 'negotiated order'. According to Strauss, the various professions and users of services find a means of working together to provide services, through the continuous development, revision, and renewal of the rules and agreements between them. While formal rules are important, the emphasis is more on informal or tacit agreements between the different professions and the users of services.

A second way of looking at the relationship between managers and health staff is through the lens of the 'professional bureaucracy' identified by Mintzberg (1980), which determines the structure within which interactions take place. The foundation for this particular structure is the 'standardization of skills'. In the case of doctors and other health professionals, their highly specialist training grants them an important degree of autonomy in their work. This autonomy is also extended to the management of their collective work. Indeed, managers often need to be professionals to gain the respect of the professional body, and ensure the authority to oversee the work. In this organizational arrangement, there is little formalization of behaviour beyond skills specialization.

These differing theories have implications for how the various professions work together, and the role of authority within this process. You can use these theories to help you think about the way health care is provided in different settings and how this might relate to the professional authority of the medical profession.

In the UK in the 1980s, non-clinical managers were introduced into the UK National Health Service to help improve the performance of the service. In this arrangement, clinicians were expected to be subordinate to managers. However, clinicians were generally unresponsive to a cadre that they perceived to be less well qualified than themselves to make decisions about the organization of health care (Llewellyn, 2001). At the same time, there was also a move to bring more clinicians into management positions. There is evidence that these clinical-management roles offered a more acceptable face of management for the general body of clinicians. We will discuss this cadre of staff that brings together the medical professional and manager, in a single role, later in this chapter.

Professions in the international context

Beyond the challenge of different cadres, doctors in all countries have had to negotiate their relationship with practitioners who subscribe to another system of medical thought, such as acupuncture or homeopathy. In some countries, biomedical doctors (sometimes referred to as allopathic) have come to dominate through sometimes fairly ruthless measures aimed at controlling and suppressing other systems. These include practices promoted under colonial administration or missionary influences in some African countries (Lock et al., 2001). However, in many countries an accommodation has been reached in which the different roles and contributions of various practitioners (traditional and allopathic) have been respected. Recognition of the important role that traditional and complementary medicine plays in many countries is captured in the 'Beijing Declaration' adopted by the WHO Congress on Traditional Medicine in November 2008 (WHO, 2008). This statement highlights the need to respect the knowledge and practices of traditional medicine, and integrate them into national systems, while also ensuring that regulations are in place to promote quality of care. In addition, as many high-income countries try to accommodate the growing use of complementary and other alternative medicine approaches in their populations, there are valuable lessons to be learned from the experience of the integration of traditional and modern scientific or allopathic medical approaches in several countries, particularly in Asia, such as China, South Korea, and India (Bodeker, 2001).

✎ Activity 5.4

Take a moment to reflect on the role of different practitioners in a country with which you are familiar. To what extent are the different medical practices integrated in this context? Does the role of allopathic medicine dominate? Given the discussion so far, can you identify some factors behind the current position of different practitioners in this context?

Feedback

There is wide variation in policy and practice relating to traditional and complementary medicine across countries. However, it is a core aspect of health services in many contexts and an important complement in many others. You may have chosen a country where there is a long tradition of multiple practitioners and where more than one medical system is officially recognized, or where single practitioners are trained in both traditional and allopathic medicine, such as rural doctors in China. Alternatively, you may have chosen a context where allopathic medicine dominates but where there is growing popularity for alternative and complementary practices, perhaps for chronic conditions, within the population. There may also be discussion around the effectiveness of different practices and how they should be funded and whether they should be funded from public money.

The role of the medical profession in society

Whether or not the public benefits from having independent professions is a widely debated issue. The following paragraphs (based on Moore, 1994) outline briefly some of the views held by social scientists on the autonomy of the medical profession.

The longest established view was that advanced by the American sociologist, Talcott Parsons, in 1939. His *functionalist* view welcomed the notion of professions, seeing the legitimation of professional status as a means of protecting patients from harm. Patients accept the authority of doctors. They trust doctors and expect them to have the highest competence. Therefore, knowledge and skills need to be guaranteed by educational standards. To protect the intimate relationship between doctors and patients, the profession needs to be granted an autonomous status, independent from state interference. Professionalism is thought to allow a more flexible response to patients' needs than tightly controlled health services. As only doctors can judge their peers, they need to have the right to discipline members who violate the code of conduct. Thus professionalism plays a beneficial role by serving both the needs of the individual and of society.

In contrast, there have been several critiques that challenge Parsons' view. In the *Marxist* view, professions are considered a middle-class privilege, mystifying and stabilizing the power of the ruling class. This was seen as part of a wider struggle between classes for economic, social, and political advantages, a struggle that was limited by the mode of production.

An alternative critique propounded by Elliot Freidson in 1974 emphasized the role of *self-interest* in the formation of professions. To him, professionalization is similar to trade unionism, a way of increasing the rewards for labour. Doctors have been particularly successful in eliminating their competitors and creating a monopoly. They have managed to keep remuneration high through market closure. And in due course, they have managed to convey the image that only members of the profession can provide services properly. In this view, professionalism is beneficial only at the expense of other occupations and to members who pursue their own interests. This view partly echoed the concerns of the liberal Irish playwright, George Bernard Shaw, who in 1911 suggested that 'All professions are conspiracies against the laity' (Shaw 1911).

More recently, the Austrian theologian Ivan Illich (1974) criticized professionalism as a way of colonizing other sectors of social life (medical imperialism) and disguising the fact that doctors produce ill health (iatrogenesis). In his view, professionalism does more harm than good. Doctors do not just provide health services but attempt to take control over other aspects of life. Examples of medical expansion include the *medicalization* of childbirth, disabilities, problems of ageing, and death. An increasing number of social problems have been handed over to the medical profession, thereby extending its authority to define what is good or wrong and barring other professions and lay people from dealing with health problems. Medical expansion is seen as a threat as it weakens individual abilities to cope with illness and hides away pain and death, which are natural parts of life.

✎ Activity 5.5

Based on what you have read so far:

1 Write down four key arguments in favour of and four against the independent status of doctors.
2 Contrast briefly the different views on independent status and compare them with your own experience in health services.

3 In your opinion, and based on your experience of a country with which you are familiar, which view best matches the role of the medical profession in practice?

Feedback

1 Some of the arguments for and against professional autonomy that you may have identified are listed in Table 5.2.
2 Although medical expansion has clearly occurred, Illich's generalizing view of the role of experts has been criticized as exaggerated and misleading (Strong, 1979). On the other hand, the functionalist view that had developed among the early writers appears to be naïve in not taking account of the self-interest of the medical profession. Freidson's view has incorporated the aspect of self-interest and given an explanation of professional power, which has been widely acknowledged.
3 Obviously your answer will depend on the professional status of doctors in your country. Opinions on professional status have changed over time, as has the power of the profession. Some of the recent publications on the subject have been less critical than those of the 1970s and 1980s (Cruess and Cruess, 1997).

Table 5.2 Arguments for and against professional autonomy

For	Against
Trust	Middle-class monopoly
Defence of individual	Medical expansion
Peer control	Dominated by self-interest
Flexibility	Lack of accountability

Threats to the medical profession

As you have seen, professiol status is not an inherent right – but is granted by society. The maintenance of the professional status accorded to medicine and other professions depends on the public's belief in the trustworthiness of those within the profession.

In recent years, some professions have been losing their position of trust within society. This is evident from the responses to surveys on the public's views on professionals such as politicians and lawyers. To date, the medical profession has generally maintained its position of trust and autonomy with the public. In the UK, this is despite a number of recent scandals in the health service. However, a number of developments within and beyond the health care system (some of which you have touched on already) are threatening the position of the medical profession:

- *Threats to monopoly*: other occupations are challenging the historical monopoly of doctors, e.g. nurse practitioners.
- *Threats to knowledge base*: a rise in consumer knowledge with access to the internet, combined with the rise of protocols and evidence-based medicine, mean that the doctor is no longer in sole possession of all the facts.
- *Threats to autonomy*: the rise of managers within the health care system is encroaching on the decision-making roles previously held by doctors.
- *Rise of consumerism*: there is a rise in shared decision-making and diminishing trust in the role of doctors as sole decision-makers. At the same time, a better understanding of rights of patients has led to increasing complaints as well as malpractice allegations. This has come at the same time as a general rise in the culture of assessment of credentials and performance.

✏ Activity 5.6

Think of the status and power of doctors in a country with which you are familiar.

- Have the status and power of doctors changed in recent years?
- What challenges have there been to medical knowledge?
- Have challenges been mounted by other professionals working in health care?

Make brief notes in response to these questions, referring to your own experience and to examples from this and previous chapters.

Feedback

You are likely to have noted that the status and power of doctors have changed in recent years. These changes, which represent threats to the profession of medicine, can also be seen as opportunities for changes in the way health services are conceived and delivered. Some of the factors which have contributed to these changes include:

1 *Managerialism*: the growing importance of managers and management processes in health care. Decisions on resource allocation are no longer left to professional autonomy. Doctors are being made increasingly accountable to those paying for health services (see the article by Relman in Chapter 1).

2 *Lay knowledge and self-help movements*: consumers have become better informed and may develop into experts in dealing with particular health problems, thereby challenging professional knowledge (see Chapter 8).

3 *Boundary disputes*: while there is medical expansion, there are also challenges from other professions taking over tasks formerly performed by doctors. For example, think of the increasing number of medicines sold without prescription by pharmacists. Nurse practitioners performing tasks formerly reserved for doctors are often seen as a challenge. Think also of psychologists or social workers dealing with drug addicts, who, it was once thought, should be exclusively treated by doctors.

4 *Medical pluralism*: the profession is increasingly divided. The interests of doctors in primary care may conflict with those in secondary and tertiary care. Sub-groups within the profession challenge traditional views. Growing specialization makes it difficult to represent the interests of all doctors. For example, in many countries instead of a single organization representing all surgeons, there are several sub-specialties with potentially opposing views.

5 *Effectiveness in question*: the issue of the extent to which medical interventions are effective has gained public attention. Many treatments have only little effect on outcomes but are promoted with professional authority. The public is increasingly aware of the limits of medicine and is becoming more critical towards medical knowledge.

6 *Ideological opposition*: doctors face opposition from other groups in society, such as other professions, social movements or parties who try to challenge the ideological monopoly of the profession. Examples include social movements fighting for consumer rights in medicine, feminist groups challenging the role of medicine in childbirth, religious groups challenging the medical definition of death and criteria for organ transplantation.

7 More general problems are those of a *loss of faith* in experts and public institutions and the *contracting role of the state*, which in some countries is taking less responsibility for health care and for protecting professional status.

These challenges do not mean that professionalism has no future or that its power is necessarily declining. There are, however, visible signs of decline in many countries. For example, in a number of countries recent health care reforms have been decided without or against the consent of the medical profession. Much of the future role of the medical profession depends on its ability to respond to these challenges. Professional organizations are increasingly aware that they need to meet the expectations of the public in order to remain trustworthy (a theme you return to in Chapter 8). And obviously they will meet these expectations more easily by placing the objective of serving the public over self-interest.

Reprofessionalization

Changes in factors that influence the nature of the profession of medicine have implications for how the profession is perceived by doctors as well as the public. Lupton (1997) coined the term 'reprofessionalization' to describe the shift in the discussion on the nature of the medical profession.

Jones and Green (2006) highlighted changes in doctors' perceptions of their role when interviewing a range of early career GPs about their work and life. Their research highlights the shift away from seeing the job as a 'vocation' to an increasing emphasis on the 'balance' between work and other aspects of life, such as time with the family or holidays. The authors note also the move away from the historically 'paternalistic' relationship between doctor and patient.

Hybrid professionals

A particular form of reprofessionalization that appears to be on the increase is that of the hybrid professional, in particular the 'professional-managerial' hybrid (Waring, 2014). Earlier in the chapter you were introduced to the idea of the clinical manager, which is one example of a hybrid professional. These hybrid roles in health, bridging the disciplines of medicine and management, present an opportunity for better communication and interaction between the medical professional and the manager (Noordegraaf, 2015). However, while the key aspects of both approaches may be embodied in a single individual, there is some evidence, at least from clinicians, that they view the management aspect of the role as supporting their clinical function, and continue to look to their clinical peers for recognition (Llewellyn, 2001).

Noordegraaf (2015) has summarized the principles that lie behind 'professionalism' and 'managerialism' from a variety of sources covering socio-political, institutional, organizational, and psychological perspectives. In his summary, Noordegraaf emphasizes the contrasting principles and values of the two roles in their pure forms. In particular, he highlights the concern in professionalism for the 'protection of professionals' and the 'primary aim of treating cases', while managerialism is more concerned with ensuring the 'proficient running of the organization' and the 'delivery of goods and services to customers'. He highlights the contrasting attributes in relation to key variables such as coordination, authority, and values, as outlined in Table 5.3.

The hybrid role embracing these different principles and values is seen as inherently 'unstable', and Noordegraaf (2015) identifies a third set of attributes for this role. However, he also suggests that there are opportunities to move beyond the instability to reach a situation where the principles of managerialism become part of the professional working practice and enhance the role of the professional, rather than undermine it – a situation he describes as 'organizing professionalism'.

Table 5.3 Professionalism, managerialism, and hybrid roles

	Professionalism	*Managerialism*	*Hybrid*
Coordination	Skills	Hierarchy	Cooperation
	Norms	Markets	Interaction
Authority	Expertise	Results	Flexibility
	Service ethic	Accountability	Reliability
Values	Quality	Efficiency	Meaningfulness
	Humanity	Profitability	Efficient quality

Source: Noordegraaf (2015).

Waring (2014) identifies the professional-managerial hybrid as one of a number of 'professional elite' roles found at the boundary between the professional and the organization. Within the health sphere, these roles place medical professionals in leadership positions that link the profession to key aspects of decision-making around health. Waring's typology identifies the six professional elite roles summarized in Table 5.4.

What is interesting about these professional elites is that their reputation appears to be contingent on both the professional and the organizational aspects of the role, and recognition is the result of approval from key stakeholders in both groups (Waring, 2014). Contrast this with the reliance on clinical peer expectations mentioned earlier for the clinical-managerial role.

Table 5.4 Typology of professional elites

Type of professional elite	*Links to*	*Role*	*Where found*
Political elite	Political process	Policy-making/Political decision-making	Professional associations Political organizations
Knowledge elite	Research organizations	Creation and dissemination of knowledge	Universities Societies of learning
Governance elite	Regulatory bodies	Regulation of work of profession	Quality standards agencies
Managerial elite	Organizational setting	Involved in day-to-day practice	Within organizations with mandate for operations
Corporate elite	Corporate markets	Influence on financial/ commercial aspects of work	Small businesses Business partnerships
Practice elite	Members of profession	Influence on specialist skills	Routine practice

Source: Adapted from Waring (2014).

These examples of reprofessionalization also suggest that the changing role of medical professionals, in particular as professional elites, is not necessarily a threat to the overall positioning of the medical profession as key influencers of health services, but rather provides them with the opportunity to continue to play an instrumental role in determining the future of the profession.

Skill mix

In the discussion so far, you have seen how a mix of health staff are employed in the delivery of health services. The particular mix of health staff within the health care system will have important implications for how services are delivered and how efficient these services are in obtaining the health outcomes desired.

The particular mix of staff in a context will be determined by various factors such as the history of the health care system and the level of economic development. You have also seen how the relative power of professions influences the roles afforded to different health workers, which will also impact on the skills mix. There is still limited evidence on the mix of skills required in a given context to achieve the best health outcomes, and in the most efficient way. What works in one context may not translate to another. What is clear is that a wide range of skill mixes is found between countries, even those with a similar level of income. This suggests that some countries are currently functioning with a below optimum mix of staff and roles (Fulton et al., 2011).

Globalization and the health worker crisis

There is a global rise in the provision of health care and health products. This growth is causing a global shortage of health workers, particularly key workers such as doctors, nurses, and midwives, although the shortages are not confined to these particular roles.

In 2006, the World Health Organization dedicated its World Health Report to the issue of the global health workforce (WHO, 2006). The report highlighted the critical shortage of health workers worldwide, and emphasized the challenges for the 57 countries where there are less than 2.3 workers per 1000 population, a threshold considered by WHO as essential to provide a basic level of health care.

One aspect of the problem is that high-income countries are increasingly looking beyond their borders to recruit staff. A substantial proportion of the workforces in high-income countries now comes from the recruitment of health staff from other countries. This is having an impact on the availability of staff in middle- and low-income countries and further exacerbating the inequalities of the global health care workforce and health outcomes. In the USA, 25 per cent of doctors are recruited externally and 60 per cent of these are from low-income countries. In the UK, the respective figures are 28 per cent and 75 per cent (OECD, 2008).

The migration of health staff, especially from low-income countries, is governed by both 'push' as well as 'pull' factors. These are illustrated in Figure 5.1. On the 'push' side, low salaries, poor conditions, and low status in many countries result in staff looking for opportunities elsewhere. On the 'pull' side, higher salaries, better conditions, and opportunities for professional development attract staff to higher-income contexts. Aspects of professional regulation and licensing, as well as immigration and bilateral agreements, can modify these push and pull factors. Some commentators argue that the 'professionalization' of medicine and nursing is also facilitating international migration, as it is promoting a common knowledge base, which can be applied across contexts.

Recognition of the damage that recruitment by high-income countries is having on the health care systems in many low-income countries has led to a global effort to monitor and contain the recruitment of health staff from low-income countries. In 2010, the WHO Global Code of Practice on the International Recruitment of Health Personnel was unanimously adopted at the 63rd World Health Assembly (WHO, 2010). This is a voluntary code and countries are encouraged to adopt it in their particular context. The Code attempts to balance the rights of individual health workers to migrate in search of better opportunities with the rights of populations everywhere to be able to access health care of a quality that ensures good

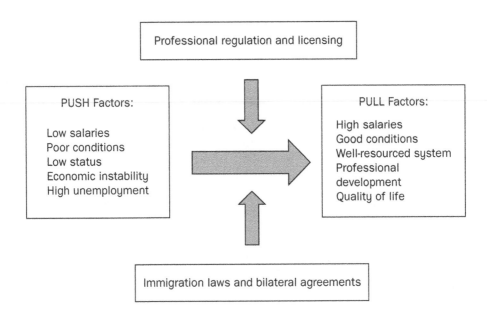

Figure 5.1 Factors affecting migration
Source: Adapted from WHO (2006).

health, by discouraging the international recruitment of health staff from countries with critical shortages. Five years on from the adoption of the Code there is some progress with countries putting in place measures to support better international recruitment of health staff, although challenges remain.

Activity 5.7

Consider once more a country with which you are familiar. Can you identify either 'push' or 'pull' factors, or both, that may encourage health staff to seek opportunities elsewhere, or that may encourage staff from other contexts to migrate to the country? What benefits or challenges do you see with this migration, either from the perspective of the health care system in this country or for those seeking health care?

Feedback

You may have identified a number of the factors outlined in Figure 5.1. If you chose a low-income country as your context, you may have listed a number of 'push' factors relating to poor remuneration or working conditions, perhaps linked to low status. The country may be going through a period of instability, either financial or political, exacerbating these factors. However, these may be counteracted by a wish to remain connected to family and friends as well as opportunities locally for professional development. Or you may have chosen a high- or medium-income country that has an expanding health sector with opportunities for health staff, including professional development, which makes it attractive to professionals from the region. Or the country may exhibit both pull factors for neighbouring countries but also be liable to push factors for health staff who see better opportunities in countries further afield.

Whatever context you chose, you will also have noted factors that are modifying these features such as whether the country has signed up to an international or regional agreement supporting health professionals, or whether there are particular restrictions and regulations governing the employment of health professionals from another country, such as language or qualification requirements.

Summary

Professionalism is a key concept in explaining the role of some occupations in health services and in society. Professional status is based on formalized training and knowledge, peer control, and a legal and ideological monopoly. The status afforded to a particular profession will be a result of the strength of these factors and dependent on public recognition of this status. In this chapter, you have considered the context of professional power and examined the different views held on professional autonomy. You have examined some of the current challenges to the medical profession and how the nature of the profession is changing, including the role of hybrid professionals, and changing perceptions of the profession by doctors themselves. You have concluded with a look at the impact of the globalization of health on health professionals.

References

Allen, D. (1997) The nursing–medical boundary: a negotiated order?, *Sociology of Health and Illness*, 19 (4): 498–520.

Allsop, J. and Saks, M. (eds.) (2002) *Regulating the Health Professions*. London: Sage.

Bodeker, G. (2001) Lessons on integration from the developing world's experience, *British Medical Journal*, 322 (7279): 164–7.

Cruess, S.R and Cruess, R.L. (1997) Professionalism must be taught, *British Medical Journal*, 315 (7123): 1674–5.

Freidson, E. (1974) *Professional Dominance: The social structure of medical care*. New York: Atherton Press.

Freidson, E. (1988) *Profession of Medicine*. Chicago, IL: University of Chicago Press.

Fulton, B.D., Scheffler, R.M., Sparkes, S.P., Auh, E.Y., Vujicic, M. and Soucat, A. (2011) Health workforce skill mix and task shifting in low income countries: a review of recent evidence, *Human Resources for Health*, 9: 1.

Illich, I. (1974) *Medical Nemesis*. London: Bantam Books.

Jones, L. and Green, J. (2006) Shifting discourses of professionalism: a case study of GPs in the UK, *Sociology of Health and Illness*, 28 (7): 927–50.

Kouta, C. and Kaite, C.P. (2011) Gender discrimination and nursing: a literature review, *Journal of Professional Nursing*, 27 (1): 59–63.

Llewellyn, S. (2001) 'Two-way windows': clinicians as medical managers, *Organization Studies*, 22 (4): 593–623.

Lock, S., Dunea, G. and Last, J.M. (eds.) (2001) *The Oxford Illustrated Companion to Medicine*. Oxford: Oxford University Press.

Lupton, D. (1997) Doctors on the medical profession, *Sociology of Health and Illness*, 19 (4): 480–97.

McLaughlin, K., Muldoon, O.T. and Moutray, M. (2010) Gender, gender roles and completion of nursing education: a longitudinal study, *Nurse Education Today*, 30 (4): 303–7.

Mintzberg, H. (1980) Structure in 5's: a synthesis of the research on organization design, *Management Science*, 26 (3): 322–41.

Moore, S. (1994) *A Level Sociology*. London: Letts Educational.

Noordegraaf, M. (2015) Hybrid professionalism and beyond: (new) forms of public professionalism in changing organisational and societal contexts, *Journal of Professions and Organisation*, 2 (2): 187–206.

Organization for Economic Cooperation and Development (OECD) (2008) *The Looming Crisis in the Health Workforce: How can OECD countries respond?* Available at: http://www.oecd.org/els/health-systems/41509236.pdf (accessed 19 April 2016).

Parsons, T. (1939) The professions and social structure, *Social Forum*, 17: 457–67.

Shaw, G.B. (1911) *The Doctor's Dilemma: A Tragedy*. London: Penguin. Reprinted 1987.

Strong, P.M. (1979) Sociological imperialism and the profession of medicine, *Social Science and Medicine*, 13 (2): 199–215.

Strong, P.M. and Robinson, J. (1990) *The NHS: Under new management*. Buckingham: Open University Press.

Waring, J. (2014) Restratification, hybridity and professional elites: questions of power, identity, and relational contingency at the points of 'professional–organisational intersection', *Sociology Compass*, 8 (6): 688–704.

Weber, M. (1947) *Theory of Social and Economic Organization*. New York: New York Free Press.

World Health Organization (WHO) (2006) *The World Health Report 2006: Working together for health*. Geneva: WHO.

World Health Organization (WHO) (2008) *Beijing Declaration*. Adopted by the WHO Congress on Traditional Medicine, Beijing, China. Available at: http://www.who.int/medicines/areas/traditional/TRM_BeijingDeclarationEN.pdf (accessed 19 April 2016).

World Health Organization (WHO) (2010) *WHO Global Code of Practice on the International Recruitment of Health Personnel*. Available at: http://www.who.int/hrh/migration/code/practice/en/ (accessed 19 April 2016).

Funding health care

6

Overview

In the previous three chapters, you have explored key inputs to health care (patients and staff) and how medical knowledge shapes them. You will now explore the other important input, finance. This chapter explains the principal revenue collection and risk-pooling mechanisms.

Learning objectives

After working through this chapter, you will be able to:

- describe the main functions and goals of health financing
- define the principles of universal health coverage
- distinguish between the principal financing mechanisms through taxes, mandatory insurance, and private payments
- describe the advantages and disadvantages of various revenue collection mechanisms
- assess the equity implications of funding decisions

Key terms

Adverse selection: When a party enters into an agreement in which they can use their own private information to the disadvantage of another party.

Catastrophic expenditure: Expenditure at such a high level as to force households to reduce spending on other basic goods (e.g. food or water), to sell assets or to incur high levels of debt, and ultimately to risk impoverishment.

Community-rated contribution: Insurance premiums that are based on pooled risk of the entire community rather than the claims experience or personal level of risk of an individual.

Cream-skimming (or cherry-picking):   When an insurance scheme enrols a disproportionate number of individuals who present a lower than average risk of ill health or high-cost care.

Moral hazard: When one of the parties to an agreement has an incentive, after the agreement is made, to act in a manner that brings additional benefits to themselves at the expense of the other party.

Pooling: The process of accumulating and managing revenue to ensure that the contributors to the pool share risks.

Progressive: A financing mechanism whereby groups with a higher income contribute a higher percentage of their income than do groups with a lower income.

Purchasing: The process of allocating funds to health care providers.

Regressive: A financing mechanism whereby groups with a lower income contribute a higher percentage of their income than do groups with a higher income.

Revenue collection: The process by which the health system raises funds from households, organizations, and external sources such as donors.

Risk-rated contribution: Insurance premium adjusted to the level of the individual's or group's risk of illness, expected future cost of health care use or past claims experience.

Universal health coverage: When all people can use the promotive, preventive, curative, rehabilitative, and palliative health services they need, of sufficient quality to be effective, while also ensuring that the use of these services does not expose the user to financial hardship.

Functions and goals of health financing

Health financing involves the three functions of revenue collection, pooling of resources, and purchasing of goods and services. The World Health Organization (WHO) defines and describes these functions as follows:

* *Revenue collection* refers to the process by which the health system raises funds from households and organizations, as well as from external sources such as donors.
* *Pooling of resources* refers to revenue accumulation and management to ensure that the financial risks associated with unpredictability of illness and unexpected health care costs are shared by all the members of the pool and spread across time and across as broad a population as possible.

- *Purchasing* refers to the processes by which pooled funds are paid to public or private health care providers in order to deliver a specified or unspecified set of health interventions (WHO, 2000).

Following the overall health system goals described in the World Health Report 2000, Kutzin (2008) notes the following health financing policy objectives:

- promoting universal protection against financial risks associated with illness;
- promoting more equitable distribution of the burden of financing the health system;
- promoting equitable use and provision of services relative to the need for such services;
- rewarding quality and providing incentives for efficiency in service delivery;
- improving efficiency in the administration of the health financing system;
- improving transparency and accountability of the financing system to the population.

This chapter discusses the revenue collection and pooling functions of health financing, while Chapter 9 discusses provider payment mechanisms as part of the purchasing function. As you are reading about various financing mechanisms in these two chapters, consider how these mechanisms compare with respect to the policy goals outlined above.

Universal health care movement

Globally, there is a growing focus on universal health coverage. In 2005, the WHO called for all member states 'to plan the transition to universal coverage of their citizens so as to contribute to meeting the needs of the population for health care and improving its quality, to reducing poverty, and to attaining internationally agreed development goals' (WHO, 2005). The World Health Report 2010, the associated declaration of the World Health Assembly, and a United Nations General Assembly resolution in 2012, reaffirmed the twin goals of ensuring access to health services plus financial risk protection, urging governments to accelerate the transition (United Nations, 2012; WHO, 2010a). Universal health coverage is currently one of the targets of the Sustainable Development Goals (Goal 3.8) (United Nations, 2015).

According to the World Health Report 2010, 'Financing systems need to be specifically designed to: provide all people with access to needed health services (including prevention, promotion, treatment and rehabilitation) of sufficient quality to be effective; [and to] ensure that the use of these services does not expose the user to financial hardship' (WHO, 2010a). The main challenge facing any financing system wishing to move towards these goals (utilization relative to need, high quality care, and universal financial protection) is to expand coverage in three dimensions: the proportion of the population with access to affordable and high quality care ('who is covered'), the range of accessible quality services available to the population in need ('which services are covered'), and the proportion of health care costs covered by the financing system ('what is covered') (Figure 6.1; Kutzin, 2013; WHO, 2010a). All countries struggle to fill the cube, and depending on where and how they start, they will travel along different paths towards universal coverage and make different choices along the three axes. You will now explore the various revenue collection and pooling mechanisms to expand the volume of the small box, which shows the health service costs that are covered from pre-paid, pooled funds.

Revenue collection

The collection process involves three elements: the sources of funding contributions, the way these contributions are structured, and the organizations responsible for collecting these contributions.

Sources of funding

Individuals and commercial companies are the main sources of funding for health care, although some funds may be channelled through non-governmental organizations and bilateral or multilateral international agencies. The main issue regarding the source of funding is the balance of

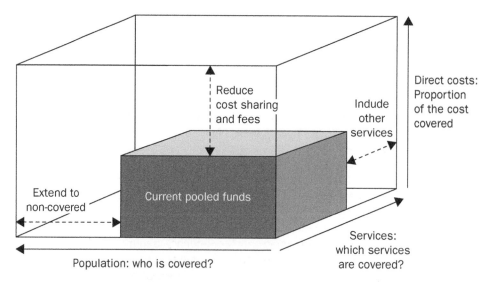

Figure 6.1 Universal coverage 'cube'
Source: WHO (2010a).

domestic and external sources; and within domestic sources, between individuals (or households) and companies (or employers) (McIntyre, 2007). The ratio of funding from individuals versus companies depends on the poverty level and income distribution of the population, the size of the formal and informal sectors, the extent to which the government wants to encourage business investment, and the ability of households/companies to make health insurance contributions. The balance between domestic and external sources is an issue for many low- and middle-income countries: while external support is often critical in meeting the health care needs of their populations, the extent of donor funding raises concerns around sustainability.

Contribution mechanisms

The main mechanisms of health care financing are government funding, health insurance, and out-of-pocket payments. Government funds include general tax revenues and external financing. Health insurance can be mandatory or voluntary ('private'). In mandatory insurance, certain population groups are legally required to adhere by the scheme. It is often referred to as 'social health insurance' or as 'national health insurance' when the entire population is covered. Insurance and tax revenue contribution mechanisms are 'prepayment' mechanisms, whereby the user contributes to health care financing through regular payments that are not related to their immediate need for health care. This is in contrast with out-of-pocket payments whereby the user pays a fee or charge at the time of receiving the health care service.

Most health systems use a mix of funding sources and collection mechanisms (Figure 6.2; OECD, 2015). In OECD countries, on average, over 70 per cent of health care spending was publicly financed (via government funds or mandatory insurance) in 2013. Central, regional or local governments financed more than 75 per cent of all health spending in Denmark, Sweden, the United Kingdom, and Italy, whereas mandatory insurance financed over 75 per cent of all health spending in the Netherlands, Czech Republic, and France. Public spending on health was below 50 per cent only in Chile and the United States. A great proportion of health spending is financed directly by households in Chile and by private insurance in the United States. While you will read about the advantages and limitations of each of the contribution mechanisms below, the desirability of one over another cannot be judged in isolation. Decisions to reduce funding through one mechanism (e.g. removal of direct payments) will automatically imply that more funds must be raised by other sources (e.g. taxation).

Out-of-pocket payments

Out-of-pocket payments take three broad forms: direct payments for services not covered by any form of prepayment (e.g. services obtained in the private sector); cost sharing (user charges) for services covered by

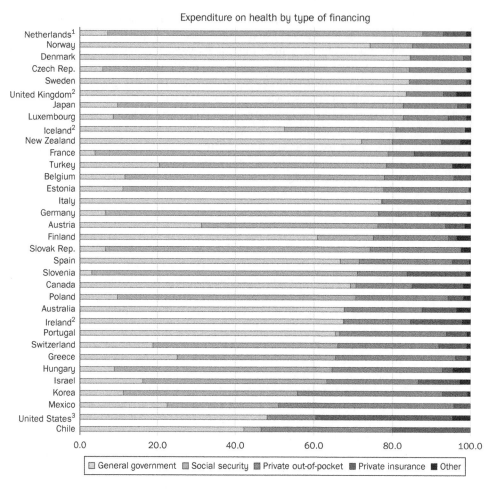

Figure 6.2 Expenditure on health by type of financing, 2013

Source: OECD (2015).

[1] The Netherlands report compulsory cost-sharing in health care insurance and in Exceptional Medical Expenses Act under social security rather than under private out-of-pocket, resulting in an underestimation of the out-of-pocket share.

[2] Data refer to total health expenditure (= current health expenditure plus capital formation).

[3] Social security reported together with general government.

the benefits package; and informal payments (also known as 'under the table' or 'envelope' payments). Very few would suggest that direct payments is a sensible method of funding health care alone unless there is no other alternative, yet some degree of out-of-pocket payments exists in most countries (Figure 6.3). Advocates of user charges argue that they can be an effective way of raising supplementary revenue for the health system, in particular when funding through taxation or mandatory insurance is inadequate or when citizens are not prepared to fund services

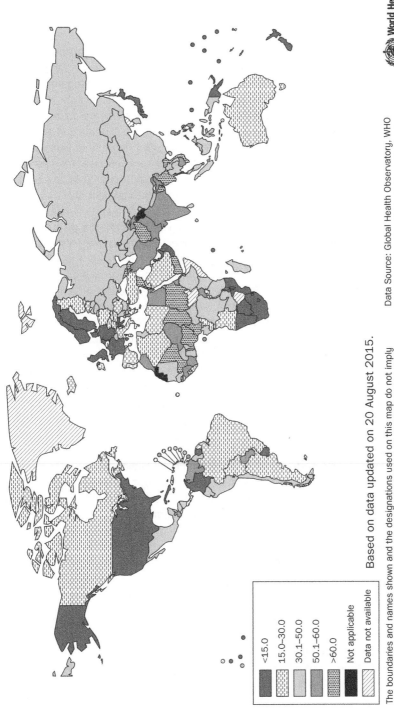

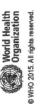

Based on data updated on 20 August 2015.

The boundaries and names shown and the designations used on this map do not imply the expression of any opinion whatsoever on the part of the World Health Organization concerning the legal status of any country, territory, city or area or of its authorities, or concerning the delimitation of its frontiers or boundaries. Dotted and dashed lines on maps represent approximate border lines for which there may not yet be full agreement.

Data Source: Global Health Observatory, WHO
Map Production: Health Statistics and
Infomation Systems (HSI)
World Health Organization

Figure 6.3 Out-of-pocket expenditure on health as a percentage of total expenditure on health, 2013

Source: WHO Global Health Observatory Data Repository (2015).

through increased mandatory contributions (Mossialos et al., 2002). The extent to which an increase in user charges impacts revenues depends on the price elasticity of demand – that is, its effect on the utilization of health services.

Out-of-pocket payments by individuals at the point of service use limits access to health care to those with the ability to pay for services. It is important therefore to consider whether cost-sharing arrangements deter excessive use of ineffective services or whether they restrict use of effective services. A review of user fees in low- and middle-income countries found that use of preventative services decreased with the introduction or increase of user fees, and increased immediately or after some time when the user fees were removed or decreased. For curative services, user fees presented a barrier to access for those groups who would be eligible to pay them (Lagarde and Palmer, 2011). Barriers to access to preventative and curative care may potentially have serious repercussions on health outcomes.

International evidence suggests strongly that high levels of out-of-pocket payments are a cause for concern, as direct payments may also have catastrophic and impoverishing effects on household finances. Households that avoid or delay seeking care might ultimately incur even higher costs, as the increased severity of their illness will require more expensive care. They might need to borrow from family or other sources with possibly high interest rates or to sell assets including livestock (McIntyre, 2007). It was estimated that about 150 million people a year face catastrophic health care costs because of out-of-pocket payments and 100 million are driven below the poverty line (Xu et al., 2007). While financial catastrophe occurs in countries at all income levels, it is greatest in countries that rely the most on direct payments to raise funds for health: there is a strong correlation between out-of-pocket payments as a share of total health spending and the percentage of families that face catastrophic health expenditure (Figure 6.4; Saksena et al., 2014).

Out-of-pocket payments can potentially be an important source of funding in low-resource settings for an individual health facility, by ensuring a reliable supply of medicines and/or by supplementing staff salaries. People may also prefer the introduction of user charges in settings where informal payments are widespread because it increases transparency. However, in addition to concerns discussed earlier, these cost-sharing arrangements are complex and expensive to administer, particularly in settings where user fee exemptions exist for poorer or chronically sick people (Mossialos et al., 2002).

Taxation

The mode of taxation, including sources (direct or indirect), types (general or hypothecated), and levels (national or local), has implications for equity, efficiency, transparency, and accountability. Taxes levied on individuals and organizations such as income tax, corporate tax, and property tax are called direct taxes. Indirect taxes are levied on goods and services (for example, value added tax, general sales tax, excise and import duties).

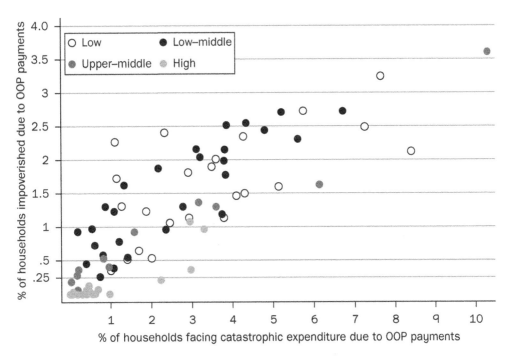

Figure 6.4 Impoverishment and catastrophic health expenditure headcount by country income. OOP = out-of-pocket

Source: Saksena et al. (2014). Licenced under Creative Commons Attribution 4.0 International (CC BY 4.0).

Direct taxes are administratively simple if formal records of income (wages or profits) are kept. In countries with a large informal sector, indirect taxes can represent the major share of tax revenue in the country.

Taxes may be collected by local, regional or central governments, and pooled in the general government budget or be hypothecated for specific purposes such as health or education. Arguments in favour of local taxation include greater transparency, improved accountability, responsiveness to local preferences, and separation of health from competing national priorities. Arguments against local taxation include domination of health care spending in local budgets and higher inequity if different tax rates are applied in different regions (Mossialos et al., 2002).

General taxation has the advantage of drawing funding from a broad revenue base and allowing for a trade-off between health and other expenditures (which ideally should reflect spending priorities of the population). However, hypothecated taxation provides a more transparent and responsive funding mechanism, which may reduce resistance to taxation and make it less susceptible to political manipulation.

Revenue generation through increasing tax funding (and to some extent donor funding) has been discussed within the context of 'fiscal space', defined as 'room or leeway within the government budget to direct resources to a specific activity that the government regards as important, without jeopardizing the sustainability of the government's overall financial situation' (McIntyre, 2007). Fiscal space is influenced by gross domestic product (GDP) per capita, the share of GDP devoted to government spending, and the proportion of total spending that is allocated to health services. In general, economic growth is associated with higher tax revenue and the proportion of economic resources devoted to government spending. Improving tax collection systems can also generate more tax revenue. For example, in Indonesia, tax revenues increased due to a simplified tax system and digitalizing paper-based processes.

Mandatory insurance

Mandatory health insurance is based on the principle of social solidarity. The most common base for mandatory insurance is contributions from the payroll (wages and salaries), which are usually split between the employer and the employee. Employee contributions create incentives for individuals to demand higher quality care and also reduce the risk of moral hazard, while employer contributions might provide incentives to encourage cost-efficient health care provision so as to keep premiums as low as possible (Borghi, 2011). The contributions could be income-related (such as a fixed percentage of income) or 'community-rated', based on the average expected cost of health service use by the entire insured group, which can also be adjusted by income levels or the number of dependents covered by the scheme.

When mandatory insurance is based on employment income only (not including other sources such as income on savings or investments), the extent of revenue generation depends on the size of the formal sector (the number of people employed), and the health care system does not have a guaranteed income. For example, a sudden increase in the level of unemployment will lead to a concomitant fall in funds available for health care. Employers might also have a disincentive to create new jobs, as the cost of employment is higher with mandatory insurance contributions. If insurance is not mandatory for the working population, employers might also have an incentive to offer part-time jobs that pay below the minimum threshold, outsource employment to self-employed contractors or create jobs in an informal 'shadow' sector (Mossialos et al., 2002).

It is sometimes argued that there is little difference between funding from direct tax and mandatory insurance – in both cases, people make compulsory income-related contributions. The presence of an independent or quasi-independent insurance fund, the clear separation of insurance contributions from tax, and well-defined rights for insured people (and the associated sense of entitlement) distinguish the two contribution mechanisms (Normand, 1999). Mandatory insurance offers other advantages relative to taxation: in contrast to funds collected by general taxation, funds collected through mandatory insurance do not need to compete with other demands on government expenditures such as defence. It is more transparent and acceptable to the public, as they know the funds will be spent on health care. Mandatory insurance, however, is more complex relative to tax-based systems and the administrative costs to collect revenue, identify beneficiaries, and reimburse their health care can be substantial. Costs might also be higher for tackling corruption and under-declaring of income (Yepes, 2005).

The World Health Report (WHO, 2010a) highlighted that all countries face challenges to revenue collection in the form of income taxes and insurance contributions from workers and their employers. Demographic transition, leading to a decline in the proportion of the working age population, has prompted high-income countries to consider alternatives to these traditional sources of revenue. In many lower-income countries, it is difficult to collect contributions, as the proportion of people in long-term employment with large employers is low, more people work in the informal than formal sector, and the share of the labour force that is self-employed or working in household enterprises is growing (World Bank, 2012). Several innovative financing options used for raising additional funds domestically were outlined in the 2010 World Health Report, and included: a special levy on large and profitable companies; a levy on currency or financial transactions; government bonds for sale to nationals living abroad; and excise taxes on tobacco, alcohol, and unhealthy food (WHO, 2010a).

Private health insurance

In private health insurance, voluntary premiums are pre-paid to a third party to cover part or all health care costs in ill health. The third party could be an independent for-profit company, a public or private non-profit organization, such as a statutory health insurance fund or a mutual association. Private health insurance can be an alternative to statutory insurance for those who can and do opt out from mandatory public insurance or are excluded from the public insurance system. It can supplement or complement mandatory systems to allow for more prompt access to health care services or to offer coverage for services that are excluded or not fully covered. Potential advantages of private health insurance include: increasing user choice, catalysing innovation and efficiency and mobilizing additional resources for infrastructure in the private as well as the public sector, and enabling relatively affluent populations to be self-financed, thereby allowing the government to target limited public resources to the disadvantaged (Mossialos et al., 2002).

Private, for-profit insurance schemes assess the risk of a person needing treatment and charge a premium based on risk factors such as age, sex, occupation, and smoking status. Given the distribution of risk in the population, this means that the actuarially fair premium is higher for older, poorer, and visibly sicker people. In practice, assessing risk is expensive and so insurance companies normally do not calculate risk for each individual, and premiums are usually group-rated (i.e. based on a calculation of the average risk of the group). Some insurance premiums may also be community-rated (i.e. based on the risk of population in a geographically defined area).

Private insurance normally results in incomplete population coverage and in general this problem is worse in poorer countries and those with a more unequal income distribution. Administrative costs of private health insurance are high, as the insurers also invest in marketing activities in order to attract members. They may also face substantial actuarial costs, particularly if contributions are risk-rated.

✎ Activity 6.1

Private health insurance markets are often regulated because of two types of market failure that exist in the health markets: risk selection and moral hazard. As you read through the descriptions and consequences of these various types of market failure, consider what measures could be used to reduce their impact.

Risk selection is usually of two kinds: adverse selection and 'cream-skimming'. *Adverse selection* arises from individuals having knowledge about their health that could be concealed from insurers: individuals with a high risk of illness and a greater need for frequent health care are more likely to enrol in a health insurance scheme. As the insurer lacks accurate information on current or future expected costs at the individual level, setting actuarially 'fair' risk-based premiums is difficult and premiums are often set in relation to the average experience of a population. Individuals with expected health care costs higher than the group average stay in the insurance pool, 'driving out' low-risk individuals. This in turn pushes the remaining individuals' premiums up, leading to further drop-outs. Insurance plans respond by *cream-skimming* (or 'cherry picking'), where they actively seek and encourage enrolment of healthy individuals. This results in incomplete and inequitable coverage, leaving disabled, sick, poor or elderly people without any insurance.

Moral hazard could be both from the provider and the consumer side. Consumer moral hazard arises because insurance reduces or in some cases eliminates the cost of health care at the point of use, resulting in overuse of health care services. For example, individuals may want to see the doctor for minor health issues because insurance will pay for it. Individuals may also participate in risk-taking behaviours, such as smoking, poor diet or inadequate exercise. Provider moral hazard arises due to the information asymmetry between the doctor and the patient. If providers are paid for their services by a third party (insurance company or government), they are not constrained by the patient's ability to pay and there is no incentive to be cost-conscious. They might also have a financial or similar incentive to increase patient consumption of health care, which can lead to supplier-induced demand.

Feedback

The primary consequence of risk selection is limited risk pooling and incomplete insurance coverage, discriminating in favour of young and healthy adults. A single pool consisting of the entire population of the country (for example, a national health service) is the obvious solution, which would eliminate this type of market failure. In settings without a compulsory, universal coverage of the population, other options that have been used to try and increase insurance coverage are educating people to take out insurance, open enrolment periods, and charging a fixed premium to everyone in a community (community rating). Differentiating individual premiums as much as possible based on risk would also theoretically reduce the rate of risk selection; however, as previously noted, this is often not feasible, as it requires accurate data and advanced tools (Hsiao, 1995).

To combat moral hazard, insurance companies often introduce cost-sharing mechanisms (such as co-payments, deductibles, and co-insurance) to place some of the financial burden on consumers. The introduction of cost sharing reduces the impact of consumer moral hazard, although there are equity implications. People in lower-income groups or those with higher utilization rates may drop out of the risk pool because of limited ability to pay the user charges. As previously noted, there is also a concern that demand for effective treatment (in addition to trivial health care) might also be reduced, with the reduction disproportionately affecting lower-income groups. The introduction of cost sharing may not reduce the impact of supplier-induced demand, as providers might switch their demand-inducing abilities from lower-income groups to those with higher ability to pay (Donaldson and Gerard, 2004). Serious health problems (of patients with no ability to pay) may be left untreated, and replaced by induced demand for care for minor health problems (of patients with ability to pay).

Community health insurance

Community health insurance is a form of voluntary health insurance that emphasizes community ownership and empowerment. Several forms of community-based financing mechanisms have been used in low- and middle-income countries, particularly in Africa and Asia since the 1990s. They are largely community initiated, owned and operated, and based on concepts of insurance and advocate solidarity at the community level. The premiums are usually flat, community-rated contributions paid monthly or annually by an individual or household.

The main advantage of community health insurance is its ability to extend financial risk protection to disadvantaged households that are often not covered by any formal insurance mechanism. With the exception of community health insurance initiatives that have been integrated into national strategies as in Ghana and Rwanda, the population coverage of the schemes has been limited. Scaling up enrolment is often challenging due to the affordability of the premiums and high poverty levels, limited awareness and understanding of the concept of health insurance, and a lack of government support. Many of the schemes are too small to function as risk pools (often limited to the village or district level) that could provide coverage for services beyond basic health care services (WHO, 2010b). Resources to sustain these schemes are also limited. Administrative costs of the community-based insurance schemes are high as in other voluntary schemes. If the contributions are income-related, determining the income status of individuals can also be difficult and costly.

Medical savings accounts

Medical savings accounts are compulsory or voluntary contributions by individuals to personal savings accounts specifically hypothecated for health care. They are based on the idea that the main issue is not the inability of families to afford health care but rather the difficulty in ensuring that the necessary funds are available at the time of need. Families or individuals have to set aside money each month and this continues until a sufficiently large fund is established. When money is spent from the fund, the family must start to save again to replenish it. These accounts may be stand-alone accounts or supplement existing insurance arrangements to provide cover for other out-of-pocket payments. Medical savings accounts originated in Singapore, where the main savings account system has two schemes to subsidize poorer and sicker people, and some more general subsidies are available for basic hospital services. They are now also used in private health insurance markets in South Africa, China, Hungary, and the United States (where they are known as health savings accounts).

Medical savings accounts do not involve risk pooling across individuals. In some settings, the fund can be passed on to the next generation upon death, which provides limited solidarity across generations but not more generally. Individuals or families are financially responsible for their lifetime health care costs. As costs for health services are borne by patients at the time of service, individuals are more likely to be aware of the price and the quality of health care and to demand fewer and more cost-effective services.

Types of collecting organizations

Central, regional or local governments, independent public bodies or social security agencies, and public or private insurance organizations collect the funds. The type of collecting organizations can have an impact on the amount and the efficiency of revenue collection (McIntyre, 2007). For example, in countries where the government has not gained the population's confidence or is not seen as accountable, tax revenues collected could be much lower than expected. Similarly, it might be preferable for a different organization to manage mandatory insurance if citizens do not trust the government to act in their best interests. For voluntary health insurance, the extent of membership will depend on how confident potential members are that their contributions will be secure and properly used (Schneider, 2005).

Pooling of funds

Pooling of funds has been defined as 'the accumulation of prepaid health care revenues on behalf of a population' (Kutzin, 2008). Risk pooling facilitates the sharing of financial risk due to unpredictability of illness across the population or defined sub-groups. Although it is difficult to predict individual health care costs, it is often possible to estimate the future health care needs of a group using epidemiological or actuarial data, and the predictability and accuracy of group health expenditures increase with the size of the risk pool (McIntyre, 2007).

Pooling occurs when funds are allocated from collection agencies to one or several pooling organizations using various allocation mechanisms. In some cases, a single organization collects and pools the funds (such as a private insurance fund); in other cases, these responsibilities may be separate. The accumulation and allocation of funds affect not only the extent to which risk protection exists, but also the equity in the distribution of health resources, and the efficiency in the organization of service delivery and in the overall administration of the health system (Kutzin, 2008). Key issues with respect to pooling of funding include the size of the population and the socio-economic groups covered by the financing mechanism, and the mechanisms used to allocate resources from pooling to purchasing organizations (McIntyre, 2007).

In some countries, the entire population is entitled to benefit from the health services funded from either taxes or mandatory insurance. In others, universal coverage is achieved with a mix of sources: often, mandatory insurance is supplemented by taxation to provide coverage for hard-to-reach groups. While the achievement of universal health coverage does not require a single scheme, it needs mechanisms to link schemes in some way. In some countries with highly fragmented health systems, a significant share of the population 'fall through the cracks' and are not covered by any of the schemes (McIntyre, 2007). You will find out more about the experiences of low- and middle-income countries that are moving towards universal coverage later in the chapter.

The second issue in pooling is about allocating central government health care resources to decentralized health authorities, which should aim for equitable distribution in accordance with health care needs and the risk of future health care costs. In some countries, there has been a shift from historically based to risk-adjusted allocation mechanisms that are designed to reduce geographic disparities in resources and promote equity of access to health care on the basis of need. These allocation mechanisms use population size, demographic composition, levels of ill health, socio-economic status, and sometimes the cost of providing health services in different areas to measure relative need. While resource allocation using needs-based formulae has been prevalent in high-income countries, it is increasingly being used in low- and middle-income settings, including Ghana, Tanzania, Uganda, Zambia, Chile, Colombia, Mexico, and Cambodia (McIntyre, 2007).

Activity 6.2

Choose a country that you are familiar with, and then explore the characteristics of the revenue collection mechanisms. You may need to obtain information from government or other sources (such as international bodies, e.g. WHO, OECD) to complete this task.

Consider the following questions:

1 What are the main sources of funding (individuals, companies, donors)?
2 What are the main contribution mechanisms (e.g. out-of-pocket, taxation, mandatory insurance, voluntary health insurance)? What is the share of public and private funding?
3 What are the pooling arrangements (e.g. is there a single pool for the whole population or multiple schemes for different populations such as the formal sector or by social groups)?

Equity in health care financing

Earlier in the chapter, we listed 'promoting more equitable distribution of the burden of financing' as a health financing policy objective. The burden of health financing is commonly measured by comparing contributions against ability to pay (usually income) and typically defined using the concepts of progressivity, proportionality, and regressivity. *Progressive financing* is a mechanism whereby groups with a higher income contribute a higher percentage of their income than groups with a lower income. *Proportional financing* is a mechanism whereby everyone contributes the same percentage of income to the funding of health care, irrespective of income. *Regressive financing* is a mechanism whereby groups with a lower income contribute a higher percentage of their income than do groups with a higher income.

A measure to assess the relative progressivity of each financing mechanism is the Kakwani Index, which compares the distribution of health care payments with the distribution of income or consumption expenditure. The index ranges from –2 to +1. A negative Kakwani Index indicates a regressive financing mechanism and a positive index a progressive mechanism. International comparisons on the distribution of the health care financing burden by funding source from European countries and the United States (Wagstaff et al., 1999), 12 Asian territories (O'Donnell et al., 2008), and Ghana, South Africa, and Tanzania (Mills et al., 2012) reveal that the relative progressivity of each financing mechanism varies by setting.

Direct taxes such as income tax are proportional or progressive, with the burden concentrated on those with higher incomes. The progressivity of income taxes tends to be lower in countries with a broad tax base, and further reduced with a lower number of tax bands and rates for each band. Income taxation by regional or local governments (such as in Denmark and Sweden) tends to be less progressive than that levied by national governments (Wagstaff et al., 1999).

For indirect taxes on goods and services, which are often charged as a proportion of the price, the burden of payment depends on consumption patterns. In most high-income countries, indirect taxes such as value-added tax (VAT) are regressive, as they are levied on a wider range of goods and services that are affordable and consumed by the majority of the population, including lower socio-economic groups. In low-income countries, indirect taxes can be a source of non-regressive financing for health care as well as contributing substantially to the total tax base (Mills et al., 2012). They tend to be progressive because the poor are more likely to survive largely on a subsistence basis (producing their own consumption items) or purchasing them from local, informal markets in low-income settings, and there are often exemption policies for commodities consumed more by the poor (Borghi, 2011). Imposing taxes on products harmful to health such as cigarettes and alcohol might be justified, as they reduce the consumption of these products, although from an equity perspective, these taxes remain regressive on average as the consumption of these products is relatively higher among low-income groups (Mossialos et al., 2002). The progressivity of general taxation depends on the relative contribution of the direct taxes and indirect taxes to revenues.

Mandatory insurance can be relatively progressive, depending on the contribution structure and the extent of population coverage. In low- and middle-income countries, insurance coverage is largely restricted to formal sector workers, with the poor making little contribution either because they are excluded from the scheme or they receive subsidized cover financed from taxation. Wagstaff and colleagues (1999) note that in some high-income countries such as Ireland, Italy, Spain, and the UK, where the contribution of mandatory insurance to total revenues was substantial in the early 1990s, it was also a progressive source of revenue due to exemptions (e.g. for pensioners, who were often among the lower-income groups) and the fact that contributions were assessed on the individual's own earnings rather than on the household's equivalent income. In the Netherlands and Germany, however, mandatory insurance was regressive due to the non-involvement of the better-off in all or part of the scheme. For high-income countries in Asia, O'Donnell and colleagues (2008) note that there is a tendency towards regressivity because the contribution of earned income to overall income (which also includes income from investments and savings) is lower in high-income groups; and mandatory insurance is only levied on earned income. Mills and colleagues note that mandatory insurance contributions are typically less progressive compared with direct tax contributions, as progressivity is likely to encourage under-reporting of salaries and remuneration in kind (Mills et al., 2012).

The progressivity of private health insurance depends on the primary purpose of private insurance cover in each country. In countries where private insurance buys cover against public sector co-payments or is taken out as supplementary cover to public insurance, these schemes tend to be progressive, as people with high incomes will more likely use private insurance and pay a greater proportion of their incomes than those from lower-income groups. Private insurance was also found to be progressive in South Africa, as it was targeted at workers in the formal sector (small population coverage, but those with relatively higher incomes than the rest of the population). In countries where private insurance is used primarily by individuals with restricted or non-existent public cover (such as the USA), it is highly regressive. Contributions to community health insurance are typically regressive due to the flat rate premium and the fact the schemes generally operate in poorer rural communities, hence posing a greater burden on the poor (Borghi, 2011).

Out-of-pocket payments were regressive in OECD countries and high-income countries in Asia. For these cases, the burden of direct payments typically falls more heavily on sick people who utilize health services more, and who are more likely also to come from deprived backgrounds. Direct payments were also regressive in the three African countries, where out-of-pocket payments are still a large share of total health care expenditure. In contrast, for several low- and middle-income territories in Asia, direct payments were found to be progressive. Relative to ability to pay, the better-off made more direct payments for health care than the poor. The poor paid less and also utilized less health care, suggesting that poorer groups cannot afford to use services and so go without health care. Therefore, the term 'progressive' here is misleading, as it refers to equitable financing but inequitable delivery of care: where everyone is expected to pay direct payments, high-income groups bear the burden but they are also the only beneficiaries of the service (McIntyre, 2007).

Progress towards universal health coverage

Many countries are now currently considering how their health financing systems can move towards or sustain universal coverage. While there is no single way to develop a financing system for universal health coverage, all forms of universal health coverage require that pre-paid funds (either tax or premium-based) are pooled, ensuring that funds from richer groups are used to some degree to subsidize the health care of poorer groups.

Activity 6.3

In the two excerpts below on revenue collection and pooling strategies for universal health coverage, William Savedoff and colleagues (2012) highlight the challenges and experiences of low- and middle-income countries, while Joseph Kutzin (2012) argues that not all paths towards universal coverage are the same. As you read through the excerpts, consider the progress made and challenges faced in your country with regards to achieving or sustaining universal health coverage.

Political and economic aspects of the transition to universal health coverage

. . . Countries of all income levels are pursuing the goal of universal health coverage. Middle-income and high-income countries that have achieved universal health coverage are still reforming their systems to address remaining inequities, improve efficiency, and contain costs. Low-income and middle-income countries that have yet to attain universal health coverage are at various stages of policy reform and resource mobilisation.

Low-income and middle-income countries face a series of challenges that high-income countries did not confront when they began to develop universal health coverage systems. The demands on health-care systems were fewer in the early 20th century because the available medical technologies were also fewer. Epidemiological challenges facing low-income and middle-income countries might also be more serious because they generally have faster-growing populations, a higher prevalence of infectious diseases, and a growing burden of non-communicable illnesses compared with countries that attained universal health coverage earlier.

However, many of these countries have learned from previous successes and failures, allowing them to make faster progress with fewer resources than did high-income countries that have already achieved universal access. Countries like Malaysia and South Korea have reached universal health coverage in two to three decades and at lower-income levels and with a smaller share of national income than the higher-income countries that preceded them. Most health spending in these middle-income countries is pooled but the mechanisms for pooling vary. For example, pooled funds in Malaysia are generated almost exclusively from general taxes whereas in South Korea they come mostly from mandatory payroll contributions.

Low-income and middle-income countries are using a wide range of strategies to achieve universal health coverage. Mexico is aiming to close coverage gaps by focusing on poor and marginalised groups. Its Seguro Popular programme provides access to health services for people who are ineligible for employment-based insurance schemes because they are self-employed, unemployed, or out of the workforce (e.g. students, children, and people who are retired). National health insurance schemes are being implemented in countries as different as Ghana, Colombia, and Indonesia. Brazil has expanded access to health care through its family health programme (Programa da Saude Familiar) and related reforms to its national Unified Health System. Thailand has dedicated public revenues to a programme that finances care, largely through public health services, for people who are otherwise uninsured. India is among those countries with the lowest share of pooled health spending, yet it is pursuing multiple initiatives to reach universal health coverage. China, which initially turned health care over to private initiative during its early market reforms, has since recognised the limitations of private financing and is seeking to expand insurance coverage through public programmes. These programmes have yielded varying degrees of success but the overall trend is favourable. They generally are pragmatic responses to a range of resilient popular pressures demanding better access to health care with greater financial protection.

This change will not, however, happen on its own. Although health spending is likely to rise in any country that has substantial economic growth and can access new medical technologies, universal health coverage will only be achieved if public policies ensure that a large share of this increased spending is pooled through a mechanism that promotes equitable and efficient utilisation of care. The exact mechanisms for pooling will depend on social processes and political action that establish the parameters for an acceptable public role in health care. In some cases, the result will be a government that primarily regulates the health-care sector, in other cases a government that finances or directly provides care. (Savedoff et al., 2012)

Anything goes on the path to universal health coverage? No.

. . . Predominant reliance on compulsory or public financing is essential for universal coverage. No country has attained universal population coverage by relying mainly on voluntary contributions to insurance schemes, whether they are run by nongovernmental organizations, commercial companies, 'communities', or governments. Compulsion, with subsidization for the poor, is a necessary condition for universality. So while it is unfortunately the case that low- and middle-income countries with poor fiscal capacity may need to explore voluntary prepayment mechanisms as an alternative to out-of-pocket payments, this is not a long-term solution. And

certainly, misplaced faith in voluntary prepayment should not provide an excuse for governments to direct public resources away from the health sector.

While public funding can come from general government revenues or compulsory 'social health insurance' contributions (payroll taxes), general government revenues are essential for universal health coverage. Even the German government injects general revenues into the system to ensure coverage for those unable to contribute. For poorer countries, the structure of the economy, with a large share of the population outside salaried employment, makes it difficult to enforce either income taxes or payroll taxes on most citizens. Thus, increasing the size of the compulsory prepaid pool of funds requires transfers from general revenues (sourced predominantly from consumption taxes (e.g. value added tax) in most low- and middle-income contexts), and the relative need for this grows in proportion to the size of the so-called 'informal sector' of the population. This further implies that moving towards universal health coverage in such contexts means moving away from the idea of a purely or even a predominantly contributory basis for entitlement and coverage.

. . . Universal health coverage goals of equitable access with financial protection require pooling arrangements that redistribute prepaid resources to individuals with the greatest health service needs. Fragmentation exists when there are barriers to this redistribution, with perhaps a worst-case scenario where there are different schemes for different social groups. For example, in most low- and middle-income countries that have initiated financing reforms with a health insurance scheme solely for the formal workforce, attention and resources are focused on already advantaged and well-organized groups, which tends to exacerbate rather than redress inequalities and leads to locking into a two-tier system.

For countries that have not yet implemented a formal sector scheme, alternatives exist. Rwanda initiated its 'community-based health insurance' system by first fully subsidizing the identified indigents from general revenues, then bringing contributions from the rest of the population into the same pools and continuing to subsidize the entire system via budget allocations for salaries and infrastructure. Kyrgyzstan and the Republic of Moldova designed a universal system from the beginning of their reforms by having a single pool for both the formal sector (from contributions) and the rest of the population (from general revenues). In a recently published review, common themes among nine African and Asian countries that had made sustained progress towards universal health coverage were both the use of tax revenues to extend coverage and the consolidation of risk pools. These examples highlight what, on reflection, should be an obvious aim for low- and middle-income countries: to use existing scarce funding sources in an explicitly complementary way. (*Kutzin, 2012*)

Summary

The principal methods of financing the health sector include general government revenue, mandatory and private health insurance, and out-of-pocket payments. The overall objective of health financing is to provide equitable and efficient health services to the population, and to minimize financial risks due to illness. Most countries use a mix of funding sources and collection mechanisms to move towards or sustain universal health coverage.

References

Borghi, J. (2011) Achieving universal coverage, in L. Guinness and W. Wiseman (eds) *Introduction to Health Economics* (2nd edn). Maidenhead: Open University Press.

Donaldson, C. and Gerard, K. (2004) *Economics of Health Care Financing: The visible hand* (2nd edn). Basingstoke: Palgrave Macmillan.

Hsiao, W.C. (1995) Abnormal economics in the health sector, *Health Policy*, 32 (1/3): 125–39.

Kutzin, J. (2008) *Health Financing Policy: A guide for decision-makers*, Health Financing Policy Paper #2008/1. Copenhagen: WHO Regional Office for Europe.

Kutzin, J. (2012) Anything goes on the path to universal health coverage? No, *Bulletin of the World Health Organization*, 90 (11): 867–8.

Kutzin, J. (2013) Health financing for universal coverage and health system performance: concepts and implications for policy, *Bulletin of the World Health Organization*, 91 (8): 602–11.

Lagarde, M. and Palmer N. (2011) The impact of user fees on access to health services in low- and middle-income countries, *Cochrane Database of Systematic Reviews*, 4: CD009094.

McIntyre, D. (2007) *Learning from Experience: Health care financing in low- and middle-income countries.* Geneva: Global Forum for Health Research.

Mills, A., Ataguba, J.E., Akazili, J., Borghi, J., Garshong, B., Makawia, S. et al. (2012) Equity in financing and use of health care in Ghana, South Africa, and Tanzania: implications for paths to universal coverage, *Lancet*, 380 (9837): 126–33.

Mossialos, E., Dixon, A., Figueras, J. and Kutzin, J. (eds.) (2002) *Funding Health Care Options for Europe*, European Observatory on Health Care Systems Series. Buckingham: Open University Press.

Normand, C. (1999) Using social health insurance to meet policy goals, *Social Science and Medicine*, 48 (7): 865–9.

O'Donnell, O., van Doorslaer, E., Rannan-Eliya, R.P., Somanathan, A., Adhikari, S.R., Akkazieva, B. et al. (2008) Who pays for health care in Asia?, *Journal of Health Economics*, 27 (2): 460–75.

Organization for Economic Development and Cooperation (OECD) (2015) Expenditure on health by type of financing, 2013 (or nearest year), in *Health at a Glance 2015*. Paris: OECD Publishing.

Saksena, P., Hsu, J. and Evans, D.B. (2014) Financial risk protection and universal health coverage: evidence and measurement challenges, *PLoS Medicine*, 11 (9): e1001701.

Savedoff, W.D., de Ferranti, D., Smith, A.L. and Fan, V. (2012) Political and economic aspects of the transition to universal health coverage, *Lancet*, 380 (9845): 924–32.

Schneider, P. (2005) Trust in micro-health insurance: an exploratory study in Rwanda, *Social Science and Medicine*, 61 (7): 1430–8.

United Nations (2012) *Global Health and Foreign Policy*, General Assembly Resolution A/RES/67/81. Sixty-seventh session. Agenda item 123.

United Nations (2015) *Transforming Our World: The 2030 agenda for sustainable development*. Available at: https://sustainabledevelopment.un.org/post2015/transformingourworld.

Wagstaff, A., Van Doorslaer, E., van der Burg, H., Calonge, S., Christiansen, T., Citoni, G. et al. (1999) Equity in the finance of health care: some further international comparisons, *Journal of Health Economics*, 18: 263–90.

World Bank (2012) *Labor Markets in Low- and Middle-income Countries: Trends and implications for social protection and labor policies*, Social Protection and Labor Policy Note #7. Washington, DC: World Bank.

World Health Organization (WHO) (2000) *The World Health Report 2000. Health systems: Improving performance*. Geneva: WHO.

World Health Organization (WHO) (2005) *Sustainable Health Financing, Universal Coverage and Mandatory Insurance*, Resolution WHA58.33. Fifty-eighth World Health Assembly, Geneva, 16–25 May 2005. Volume 1. Resolutions and decisions. Document WHA58/2005/REC/1. Geneva: WHO.

World Health Organization (WHO) (2010a) *The World Health Report 2010: Health systems financing: The path to universal coverage*. Geneva: WHO.

World Health Organization (WHO) (2010b) *Community Health Insurance and Universal Coverage*, Technical Brief Series, Brief #6. Geneva: WHO.

World Health Organization (WHO) Global Health Observatory Data Repository (2015) *Health Expenditure Ratios, All Countries, Selected Years: Estimates by country*. Available at: http://apps.who.int/gho/data/node.main.75 (accessed 19 April 2016).

Xu, K., Evans, D.B., Carrin, G., Aguilar-Rivera, A.M., Musgrove, P. and Evans, T. (2007) Protecting households from catastrophic health spending, *Health Affairs (Millwood)*, 26 (4): 972–83.

Yepes, F. (2005) Corruption in the health sector: The Colombian experience, in S. Nitayarumphong, A. Mills, Y. Pongsupap and V. Tancharoensathien (eds) *What is Talked about Less in Health Care Reform?* Nonthaburi, Thailand: National Health Security Office.

SECTION 3

Processes of health care

Need, demand, and use

Overview

Having looked at the inputs to care, you will now examine in more detail the processes (or activities) of health care. In this chapter, you will explore the dimensions of need, the roles of illness behaviour and clinical judgement, and their relationship with service use. You will study various ways of measuring health services activity, the reasons behind variations in care, and explore the question of the extent to which use reflects need.

Learning objectives

After working through this chapter, you will be able to:

- understand concepts of need, demand, and use
- distinguish between different types of need
- outline the process of assessing the health care needs of populations
- understand the causes of variations in utilization rates
- conceptualize the relationship between use and need
- distinguish between different categories of care

Key terms

Clinical or professional judgement: The decision taken by a clinician as to whether or not a patient has a normative need.

Demand: Expressed need for health services.

Inverse care law: The observation that availability of care appears to be inversely related to need.

Random variation: Statistical differences that occur by chance and are inevitable when counting events.

Relative need: Comparison between needs of individuals with similar conditions or between needs of populations living in similar areas.

> **Systematic variation:** Statistical differences that cannot be accounted for by the inevitable random variations that occur when counting events.
>
> **Use:** Utilization of health services that are actually provided.
>
> **Utilization rate:** A measure of health service use.

A conceptual model of need, demand, and use

The following model, which is represented diagrammatically in Figure 7.1, will help you to understand better the relationship between need, demand, and use.

The process starts with the population, some of whom have a subjective view that they have a *need for health*, which, as you saw in Chapter 3, is known as *felt need*. Depending on their personality, circumstances, and beliefs, they may approach formal health services and make a *demand* (also referred to as *expressed need*). Alternatively, they may decide that the problem is not serious, will resolve without treatment or can be dealt with by lay care. Their felt need has not gone away but has not been turned into a demand for formal care. As you can see, people's *illness behaviour* will be a key determinant of the level of demand for formal care.

The next step is determined by the health care professional's reaction to the person's demand. *Clinical or professional judgement* determines whether or not the person's need for health is also a *need for health care*. If the clinician feels there is an appropriate and effective intervention available that the person could potentially benefit from, the clinician will confirm a

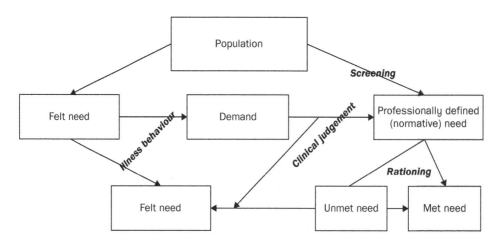

Figure 7.1 A conceptual model of need, demand, and use

normative need exists. If not, the person will be discharged from formal care, albeit that they still have a need for health.

Those deemed to have a normative need will either be treated (*met need*) or they may have to wait until resources allow treatment (*unmet need*). This is one form of *rationing*. Care may also be rationed on the ability to pay such that those who cannot afford it will not be able to turn a felt need into a demand. Some normative need may never be met, if the necessary service does not exist, so some people will continue with their felt need.

Returning to the population, there is one other circumstance to consider. There will be some people who feel fine and have no felt need but are harbouring the early stages of a disease (referred to as pre-symptomatic) or are at high risk of developing a disease. Most countries have some screening programmes to try and detect such people. Those identified through screening will have a normative need but no felt need.

🖊 Activity 7.1

These concepts are illustrated by the following examples, which describe four patients. Consider each and describe the situation using the terms you have been introduced to above.

1 Patient A presents with abdominal pain. The surgeon diagnoses appendicitis and recommends an operation, appendectomy.
2 Patient B has osteoarthritis of the hip and wants the joint to be replaced. The doctor approves of the demand and puts her on a waiting list.
3 Patient C has flu caused by a virus and demands drug treatment. There is no effective pharmaceutical intervention from which the patient could benefit.
4 Patient D is thought by his doctor to be suffering from depression and could benefit from treatment but the patient is unconcerned.

Feedback

1 Clinical judgement deems there is a need for health care. Felt need is congruent with normative need. The surgical intervention means Patient A's need is met.
2 Felt need and normative need are congruent but due to rationing, need is not immediately met. It may be turned later into a met need.
3 There is a felt need but clinical judgement deems that there is no normative need. Clinical judgement did not substantiate the demand. The patient's felt need (for health) remains.
4 There is no felt need and so there is no expressed need. However, there is a normative need.

Need

As you have seen above, it is important to distinguish between different types of need. Recall that *felt need* (*the need for health*) is subjective, determined by the individual's perceptions of their need for health. Measurement of the extent of felt need in a population requires population surveys of self-assessed health, and it is the focus of most epidemiological studies.

Normative need (*the need for health care*) depends on the judgement of professionals. The professional view is that to benefit from care, there needs to be an effective intervention. Normative need varies over time and with the health care system. Often you will see international differences in the recommended policies by professional organizations, based on the same scientific evidence. These variations largely reflect the differences in availability of resources and health care expenditure.

Differences in views of normative need affect whether or not whole services are provided. In a comparison of several European countries (including France, Switzerland, Germany, the Netherlands), it was found that while some services are included in publicly funded services everywhere (such as medical care, nursing home care, prescription drugs), other services are more controversial and not universally provided (such as dental care, home help, spas, chiropractic) (Polikowski and Santos-Eggimann, 2002).

The third type of need is *unfelt need*. This depends on the existence of pre-symptomatic disease, which is not perceived by the individual.

In addition, there is the concept of *relative need*. This refers to the level of need of a population rather than a single individual. It is based on a simple comparison of the level of provision and use of a service in similar populations. If area A provides more care than area B, the latter may be said to have a relative need for more services. Such a judgement takes no account of whether the appropriate level of service is that provided in area A or area B. It assumes that more care is the correct policy.

Demand

Demand arises when the need for health leads to action in search of care. It depends on felt need, illness behaviour, and the supply of services.

As you have seen, whether people take action to seek care when they have a need for health depends on their perception of diseased status and cultural factors (see 'What is disease?' in Chapter 3). Of course, these needs may not be expressed to formal carers. John Last, an Australian doctor, addressed this question in the early 1960s. He concluded that there was a 'clinical iceberg', as illustrated in Figure 7.2. It suggests that a large proportion of need lies submerged below the surface and is not presented to formal carers.

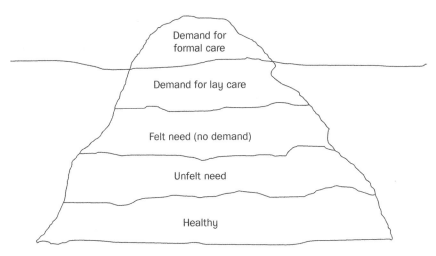

Figure 7.2 The clinical iceberg
Source: Last (1963).

✏ Activity 7.2

John Last concluded that some (or all) of the submerged iceberg should be hauled up above the surface so that more people receive formal care. For each of the segments of the submerged iceberg, do you think such advice is well founded?

Feedback

With the benefit of hindsight, Last's argument seems to be less convincing than when he made it in 1963. There are several reasons for this, some of which you may have thought of:

1   'Demand for lay care' may be for conditions that do not require formal care such as many musculoskeletal conditions or minor psychological problems. Last's argument implies that people in this category would do better in the hands of formal carers than they are doing with lay carers. There is little evidence to support this.

2   Those with a 'felt but unexpressed need' may have made a considered decision to do nothing about their problem. To suggest such people ought to be demanding formal care is to encourage supplier-induced demand. It is an example of the innate tendency of formal carers to try and 'medicalize' people (as you saw in Chapter 3).

3 Those with an unfelt need can only be detected through screening. While many screening programmes have been demonstrated to be effective, many others remain controversial because the benefits to some people are outweighed by the harm and cost to others.
4 The 'healthy' should be encouraged to stay away from formal care!

Demand for services (and whether demand is turned into use) also depend on supply of services, which includes the availability of resources and clinical judgement. Clinical judgement can encourage or discourage demand for a service. For example, if a surgeon is not interested in a particular condition or operation, potential patients will be discouraged from seeking care. Similarly, a clinician with a special interest can attract additional patients (often referred to as *supplier-induced demand*). Resource availability and clinical judgement are interrelated: if the number of beds in a hospital is doubled, the judgement of the clinicians may change such they now admit patients who previously were not admitted. In other words, the criteria that define normative need are altered.

You should be aware that clinical judgement may vary between professionals and over time, and variations in clinical decisions are common. A simple example appeared in a British newspaper following a journalist visiting five dentists for a routine check-up. While one dentist's judgement was that nothing further needed to be done, the other three recommended dental care costing £16, £198, and a staggering £1700! (Collinson, 2010). Often these variations reflect an underlying lack of agreement as to what is the best form of treatment. However, it also may reflect other, less justifiable reasons. Professionals take decisions in the light of what is best for:

- themselves (aspiration for income; enjoyment of a satisfactory practice; desire for approval from their peers);
- the patients (using every conceivable treatment regardless of cost);
- third parties/society (keeping to cost-containment policies of their employers and those paying for care; avoidance of their perceived risk of litigation).

All of these are legitimate interests, which professionals need to keep in balance. Most health services problems are a result of a lack of balance between these three interests.

Activity 7.3

Doctors routinely assess the health needs of individual patients but how can they assess the health care needs of groups of patients or whole population? The article that follows on needs assessment by two public health doctors, Andrew Stevens and John Gabbay, examines some of the problems of needs assessment of populations and applies the needs, demand, and use framework used in this chapter. While reading the article, focus on who is involved in needs assessment and whose view should be considered to determine needs.

When you have finished reading, make fairly detailed notes in response to the following questions, drawing on what you have read.

1   Which professions and which organizations are involved in assessing population needs in your country? Think, for example, of needs assessment for services for AIDS patients, the mentally ill, or mothers and children.
2   How would a needs assessment based on felt need differ from one that focuses primarily on normative need? Think of potential conflicts between the views of professionals and of the public, and the impact of both views on change of health services.

Needs assessment needs assessment . . .

A working definition of needs

Information about deprivation or mortality may tell us something about the need for health, but of itself says little about the need for health care. The two should not be confused. The need for health is related to the overall aim of a healthier population, but the need for health care is the current focus of needs assessment to improve the effectiveness of health services.

Therefore, in the present context, 'need' can be defined as the ability to benefit in some way from health care. After all, there can be no rational need for either an individual, or a population, to receive an item of care that confers no benefit. The ability of the population to benefit from health care depends on two things: the number of individuals affected, i.e. the incidence and prevalence of the condition under question, and the effectiveness of the services available to deal with it. Ideally, it will also take into account aetiological and other factors that are likely to influence the natural history of the disease or interfere with an intervention, but which are outside the scope of health services provision. Therefore, assessing needs must, at the very least, require us to have detailed information about those aspects of each condition for which we are considering the provision of preventive, diagnostic, therapeutic, rehabilitative and/or continuing care. Conditions will have to be defined quite clearly, and often sub-divided by severity, because each form of care may have only very narrow indications. Therefore despite the simple definition of needs, there is a very large task, which is compounded by the interaction of need with demand and supply.

'Need', 'demand' and 'supply'

The distinction between need, demand and supply is well established, but further exploration is required in order to clarify the approach to 'needs' in service contracts, and to the information sources currently used for needs assessment.

. . . Need, demand and supply overlap. This means that there are eight potential fields – including the external Field 8 where a potential service is not needed, demanded or supplied [see Figure 7.3]. A health care intervention for any specific condition will fit into one of these fields. Examples for the content of each field abound: in Field 1, an example of what is needed, but neither supplied nor – on balance – demanded, might be a local proposal to increase substantially the rehabilitation facilities. Field 3 might include routine caesarean sections on women with a history of a

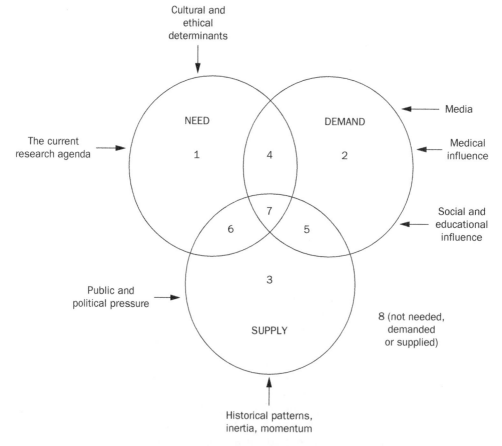

Figure 7.3 Need, demand, and supply: influences and overlaps

Source: Stevens and Gabbay (1991).

previous section, which is neither demanded nor needed but continues to be supplied. In Field 5, an example of a service that is demanded and supplied, but not needed, would be the prescription of antibiotics for uncomplicated viral upper respiratory tract infection. Any useful assessment of needs will require not only an analysis of the relationship between need, demand and supply for the many conditions under consideration, but an attempt to see how the three can be made more congruent. Since all the fields are subject to change, the ideal would be to bring them closer together so that everything that is supplied is needed; and recognised as such by everyone. Health services would be more effective and also more efficient if as many services as possible were in Field 7.

Information sources

The model [see Figure 7.4] may be used to demonstrate what information sources really tell us about needs in the context of supply and

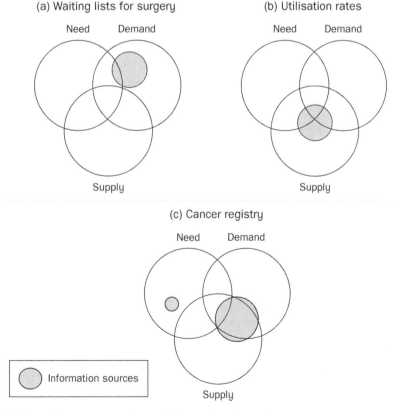

Figure 7.4 Information sources and need, demand, and supply
Source: Stevens and Gabbay (1991).

demand. The health service [in most or all countries] has always based its descriptions of need, however defined, on a variety of information sources. These include demographic data from the census, surveys on health status and on the views of patients, hospital utilisation rates, waiting lists, morbidity rates from registers and survey data, and (to a minor extent) studies on the effectiveness of interventions. Most of the routine sources are notoriously inaccurate, but even if they were perfect, substantial problems would remain, not least because there are no generally agreed definitions of 'morbidity', or 'health problems', that will allow the unambiguous interpretation of the current diagnostic categories used in routine statistics.

Strictly, the assessment of needs, defined as the ability to benefit from care, would rely most heavily on detailed knowledge of morbidity rates and studies of effectiveness, which are relatively rare. However, since all the available routine information sources are being used in the current attempts at needs assessment, it is worth reviewing what they tell us. A few examples will suffice to highlight their limitations as measurements of need:

i   *Waiting lists for surgery describe demand, which may be stimulated by supply and which may or may not be needed [see Figure 7.4a].*
ii *Utilisation rates describe supply that may be either demanded, or needed, or both, or neither. Dental extractions, for example, may be performed for good clinical indications on people who prefer not to have them (a need not demanded), or at the patient's request when there is no clinical indication (a demand not needed), or even unscrupulously for profit (supplied, but neither demanded nor needed) [see Figure 7.4b].*
iii *Even morbidity information may tell a variety of stories. Cancer registry information does not in itself clarify the need for the treatment of, say, bronchial carcinoma, which can entail services that cover every combination of need, supply and demand [see Figure 7.4c]. For example, where pneumonectomy does not alter a patient's prognosis, it is part of the supply that is not needed, but other forms of care, including preventive measures or continuing care, may confer benefit but be inadequately supplied, while others will still be demanded whether needed or not. Hence morbidity data do not clarify the need for health care, unless complemented by a detailed knowledge of the effectiveness of services.*

The current agenda

Clearly, there are difficulties both with the meaning of need and with the value of the information available to assess it. Thus, although an epidemiologically sound assessment of needs is crucial to the development of health services, it will take a long time to produce.

... Firstly, there already exists a rough and ready epidemiological view of many needs, which should not be rejected on the grounds of its scientific impurity. For example, the shortcomings of the broad balance of care for ischaemic heart disease or child surveillance are already well enough known. A second standpoint ... is to measure relative provision, which, without any other evidence, can provide clues to areas where changes are warranted. Thirdly, the preferences of local general practitioners are another powerful mechanism for improving the congruence between service contracts and local health needs ... The same can be said of consumer opinions, which are canvassed by many health authorities as a step towards matching services to local demands, although often with the emphasis on the quality rather than the scale of services ... Finally, there will always be managerial priorities dictated by central policy and modified by local considerations. The call for day surgery is a good example ...

Conclusion

The very difficult task of assessing health needs will be aided by a clear distinction between need, supply and demand. This is important because successful adjustments to health care delivery will depend on how far need, supply and demand are made congruent. This success will in turn ultimately depend on a focused epidemiological research programme, but in the short term much can be done with the available tools.

Reprinted from Stevens, A. and Gabbay, J. (1991) Needs assessment needs assessment ..., *Health Trends*, 23:20–3. Crown Copyright material is reproduced with permission of the Controller of HMSO and the Queen's Printer for Scotland.

Feedback

Now compare your notes with the feedback below:

(1) There are immense organizational and technical problems in assessing the health care needs of the whole population. Most services are determined without information on population need. Ministries of health may have planning units or there may be joint commissions between government or social insurance organizations and the medical profession. Ideally, needs assessment should be based on epidemiological data from research studies, which are applied to specific populations. If these are not available, assessing relative need may be the only feasible technique. Note that it is important to integrate professional views with the views of the public to increase accountability for the decisions.

Coordinating different professions and organizations as well as public views can be difficult. It may well be that the different groups do not take account of each other's views. Where the medical profession is involved in needs assessment, decisions are likely to be influenced by patients' demand and the interests of doctors.

(2) An approach based on felt need would reflect the views of the public, while a normative needs approach is based on professional views. Focus on felt need could make services more responsive to the public but could result in services being provided that are not cost-effective. Formal services aim to meet the need for health care rather than the need for health.

Use

You will now explore how to measure use of health services and examine why utilization rates vary, both internationally and within countries.

Utilization rates can either be *service-based* or *population-based*. Service-based rates use the number of people receiving care (such as the number of pregnant women cared for by the community midwife) as the denominator. Population-based rates use the general population as the denominator. The following activity asks you to reflect on the range of measurements of service use.

Activity 7.4

Based on your experience, give examples from primary care and hospital care of some service-based and population-based rates.

Feedback

Your response will reflect your experience.

1 Service-based rates (i.e. with no reference to the size of the population served):

- *Primary care* – number of referrals to secondary care per primary care consultation; number of home visits per community nurse; ratio of proprietary to generic prescribing.
- *Hospital care* – operations conducted as day care per 100 total (day care plus inpatient) operations; proportion of patients in intensive care units.

2 Population-based rates

- *Primary care* – immunization coverage.
- *Hospital care* – hospitalization rates.

Variation in utilization rates

The following examples illustrate the extent to which variations in utilization exist around the world. Regardless of health care system, such variations are a universal feature.

Service-based rates

1 In the 1990s, the number of referrals to hospital specialists made by general practitioners (GPs) in Finland varied from 7 per 1000 consultations for the 20 per cent of GPs with the lowest referral rates to 115 per 1000 for the 20 per cent of GPs with the highest rates (Vehvilainen et al., 1996). Similar variation can be seen across 211 GP practices in England and Wales, for which referral rates varied from 2.4 per cent to 24.4 per cent (Sullivan et al., 2005).
2 Proportion of people with stroke admitted to an acute stroke unit within 4 hours of arrival to hospital in England in 2013 varied nearly four-fold between districts, from 22 per cent to 85 per cent (NHS England et al., 2015).
3 Across OECD countries, the share of cataract surgeries carried out as day cases ranged from less than 40 per cent in Lithuania, Poland, Hungary, and the Slovak Republic to over 95 per cent in the Nordic countries, the Netherlands, and Spain in 2012 (OECD, 2014).
4 The ratio of proprietary to generic antidepressant (SSRI and SSNIs) prescriptions for Medicare patients for 306 referral regions in the USA ranged from 15 per cent to 51 per cent in 2008 (Donohue et al., 2012).

Population-based rates

1 Haemophilus influenzae type b (Hib) vaccine had been introduced in 192 countries by 2014. Global coverage with three doses of Hib-containing vaccine is estimated at 56 per cent in 2014, reaching 90 per cent in the Americas, but only 21 per cent and 30 per cent in the Western Pacific Region and in the South-East Asia Region respectively (WHO/UNICEF, 2015).
2 Hospitalization for ambulatory care-sensitive conditions (specific long-term conditions such as diabetes, epilepsy, and high blood pressure, which should not normally require hospitalization) is widely used as an indicator of access to and quality of primary care. In 2013–14, emergency admission rates for ambulatory care-sensitive conditions ranged from 184 to 1586 admissions per 100,000 population across districts in England (Figure 7.5; NHS England et al., 2015).
3 Among 132 countries, the proportion of babies born by caesarean section varied from 1.4 per cent in Niger to 55.6 per cent in Brazil in 2012 (Ye et al., 2016).

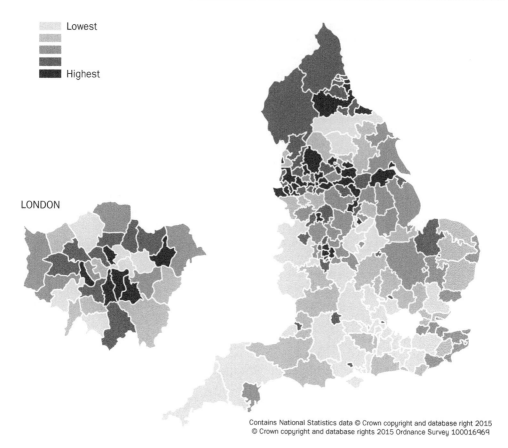

Figure 7.5 Emergency admission rates for ambulatory care-sensitive conditions
Source: NHS England et al. (2015).

4 The proportion of births attended by 'skilled health staff' in 2010–14 varied from 22 per cent in Chad and 34 per cent in Bangladesh, through 59 per cent in Côte d'Ivoire and 68 per cent in Ghana, to 83 per cent in Indonesia and 100 per cent in Cuba, according to the World Development Indicators (World Bank, 2015).
5 Across OECD countries, age-standardized rates of hysterectomy were three times higher in the USA and Canada than in Spain or Ireland in 2008 (OECD, 2014).

What causes variations in use?

The finding that the use of health care varies between areas and over time is not, in itself, either a good or a bad thing. We first need to understand why variations occur. The following activity encourages you to reflect on patient- and health service-related factors that might influence utilization at various levels of health care.

✎ Activity 7.5

Suppose the manager of a district hospital has observed that a certain operation is being performed more frequently than in the past and asks you to investigate possible causes. Draw on what you have learnt so far in this book to annotate the figure below with all the possible patient-related (demand) and health service-related (supply) factors that might influence:

- the presentation rate to general practitioners
- the referral rate to the district hospital
- the intervention (surgical) rate.

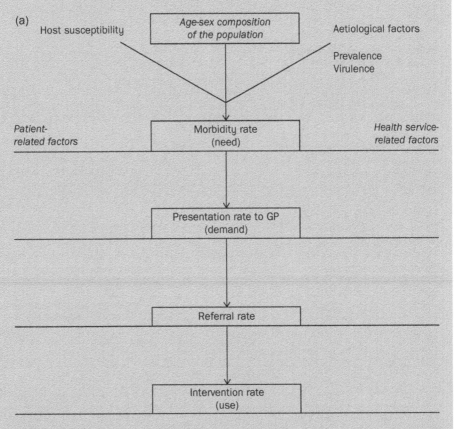

Figure 7.6a Activity

Feedback

Compare the factors on your completed figure with those shown on the figure below.

As you can see in Figure 7.6b, some factors appear more than once. Clinical judgement may vary in the different settings, as may patients' concerns, payment methods, and costs. Note that travel costs, particularly in low-income countries, are an important factor in access to care, adding to the direct costs borne by the patient.

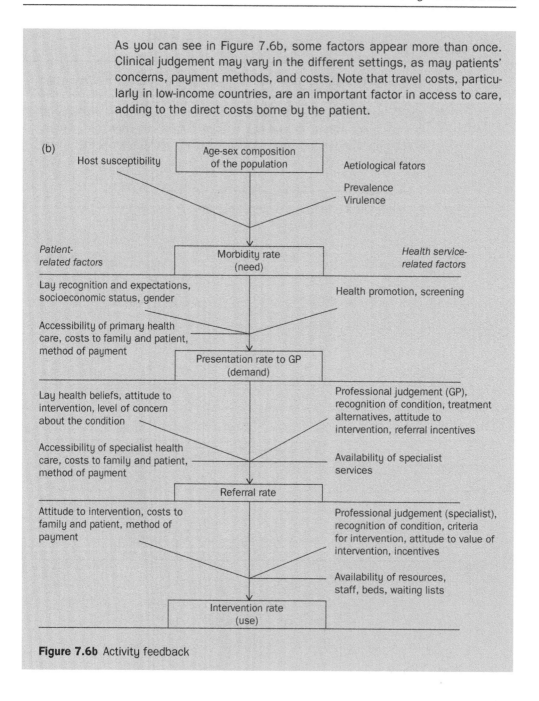

Figure 7.6b Activity feedback

There are three categories of factors you need to consider when trying to explain variations in care: statistical factors, demand-side factors, and supply-side factors.

Statistical factors

Statistical factors include data quality and random variation. Common data quality issues that need to be checked, reported and, if possible, corrected are incomplete data collection and inconsistent data specification, including clinical coding. You need to ensure that information on all cases under consideration are accounted for and accurately reported in the data sources, and that data quality is comparable across providers or regions.

Observed differences may also be due to chance (random variation), which could be taken into account by using standard statistical probability tests. Statistical differences in observations resulting from experimental or other situations that cannot be accounted for by the inevitable random variations are called 'systematic variations'.

Demand-side factors

Demand-side factors that contribute to variations in use include need and illness behaviour. Demographic composition (age and sex) and frequency of disease vary across populations and have an impact on overall morbidity rate (need). Illness behaviour varies with cultural attitudes and socio-demographic characteristics.

Analysis of variations in health care utilization must take account of the socio-demographic factors affecting need. Almost all analyses adjust for sex and age distributions, as the data are likely to be routinely available. The relationship between age and utilization rates tends to follow a pattern whereby health care is used more in the first years of life and by the elderly. An example of this can be seen in Figure 7.7, which shows how the level of health care expenditure for women varies with age in the Netherlands (Mackenbach et al., 2011).

Socio-economic status is another determinant not only of morbidity and mortality but also of health care utilization. In general, more deprived or poorer areas suffer higher rates of illness than more affluent areas, and therefore areas of higher deprivation are expected to have higher rates of health care use.

A study that compared mortality and self-assessed health by socio-economic groups among 22 countries in Europe found that, in almost all countries, the rates of death and poorer self-assessments of health were substantially higher in groups of lower socio-economic status (Mackenbach et al., 2008). Socio-economic status is associated with the utilization of specific procedures, primary care versus specialist care, elective versus emergency services, with the strength of association reflecting the differences in need, as well as access to services. In a study of 21 OECD countries, the number of physician visits was higher for patients with higher income levels (sometimes called pro-rich inequity) in over half of the countries, with the degree of inequity highest in the USA and Mexico. There was

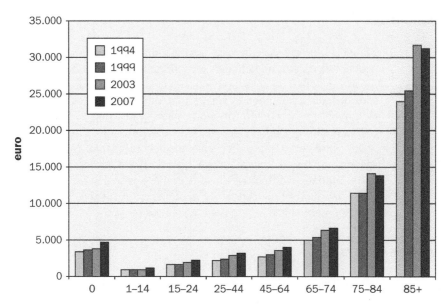

Figure 7.7 Variations in health care expenditures by age groups
Source: Mackenbach et al. (2011). With permission of Springer.

no evidence of inequity in primary care visits across income groups for most countries, and where it occurred, it was pro-poor. However, in all countries and after adjustment for need, patients with higher income levels were more likely to visit – and to visit more frequently – specialist care, with largest pro-rich inequity for specialist visits in Portugal, Finland, and Ireland (van Doorslaer et al., 2006).

In England, a review of evidence from studies on utilization of the NHS concluded that while the distribution of primary care utilization is broadly equitable across income levels, the use of specialist treatment and, in particular, use of outpatient care was pro-rich (higher relative to need among higher socio-economic groups) (Dixon et al., 2007). In Spain, a study using data from six National Health Surveys from 1993 to 2006 concluded that individuals who had manual occupations were more likely to visit primary care and emergency services more than those with non-manual occupations. In contrast, those from non-manual classes were more likely to use specialized services (and in particular dental services) more frequently (Palència et al., 2013).

There are various approaches to assess the relationship between use and need. One of the first attempts to calculate a *use/need ratio* was conducted in the UK in 1978 (Le Grand, 1978). The level of need for each socio-economic group was determined from a population survey of self-assessed health and the level of use was calculated using data from the health service. This showed that health care use for the most affluent socio-economic group was 41 per cent higher than for the least affluent group, taking into account the greater level of need in the least affluent group.

Activity 7.6

Thinking about the concepts of need discussed in this chapter, what do you think was the major limitation of such a comparison?

Feedback

The measure of need was that of felt need. Health services should be provided and used according to normative need that takes into account whether or not a cost-effective intervention exists.

An attempt to compare use and need using a proxy measure of need was carried out by Nick Black and colleagues (1995). They looked at coronary revascularization procedures, which are common in high-income countries for coronary heart disease. The normative need in the population for these procedures was determined by the standardized mortality ratio (SMR) for coronary heart disease. Age-sex standardized revascularization rates were inversely correlated with SMRs. In other words, higher intervention rates were associated with districts with lower SMRs (i.e. lower need). A similar relationship between socio-economic status and the use of coronary surgery was observed in Rome, Italy (Ancona et al., 2000). The authors found that the most affluent men had surgery at the rate of 14.1 per 100 cases of coronary heart disease compared with only 8.9 per 100 among the least affluent. These findings were similar to those of Le Grand in 1978: the use of surgery was higher in districts with lower levels of need.

A second approach to assessing the relationship between use and need is to compare the levels of need among patients who actually receive services. If use reflected need, those using particular services would have conditions with similar levels of severity. Neuburger and colleagues (2012) described how disease severity and duration were associated with age, sex, ethnicity, and socio-economic status in patients undergoing hip or knee replacement surgery in England in 2009–10. They hypothesized that if there were inequalities in the use of health care, they would expect to see differences in disease severity and in duration of problems between patients at the time of surgery. They found that patients who were socio-economically deprived had more severe hip and knee problems at the time of surgery, and more often long-standing problems, suggesting that these patients tend to have surgery later in the course of their disease.

It is possible that such differences reflect patients' preferences for care. However, studies with data that can account for illness behaviour to explain variations in care are limited in number. Hawker and colleagues (2001) used population-based mail and telephone surveys to assess whether area rates for arthroplasty reflected five-fold differences in levels of patient demand in Ontario, Canada. The demand-side factors considered in the study included both the potential need for and individuals' willingness to undergo arthroplasty. They found that among patients with severe arthritis, only 9 per cent in the low-rate areas and 15 per cent in the high-rate areas were willing to undergo joint arthroplasty. The study demonstrated that observed geographic differences in rates were explained in part by patients' willingness to undergo the procedure. Furthermore, there was a wide gap between the demonstrable need for the procedure and patients' willingness to undergo the procedure. As a result, estimates of need for the procedure, once adjusted for willingness, were much lower than estimates based on need alone.

Supply-side factors

Supply-side factors include variations in the availability and organization of resources (such as the number and distribution of facilities and staff, amount and method of funding, service configuration) and clinical judgement. In 1971, Julian Tudor Hart, a GP working in Wales, recognized that service availability often appears to be inversely related to need. In his classic essay, he coined the 'inverse care law' as:

> In areas with most sickness and death, general practitioners have more work, larger lists, less hospital support, and inherit more clinically ineffective traditions of consultations than in the healthiest area; and hospital doctors shoulder heavier case loads with less staff and equipment, more obsolete buildings and suffer recurrent crises in the availability of beds and replacement staff. These trends can be summed up as the inverse care law: that availability of good medical care tends to vary inversely with the need of the population served. (Hart, 1971)

One of the earliest studies of the relationship between clinical judgement and variations in surgery rates was in the 1930s by a British paediatrician, J. Alison Glover, who identified a four-fold variation in tonsillectomy rates among school districts. He observed that the key decision-maker regarding the need for tonsillectomy was a single physician, the school's health officer, and after ruling out a number of environmental and illness-related factors, he hypothesized that the major source of variation in the tonsillectomy rates was the difference in the medical opinion of the health officers (Glover, 1938). The evidence that Glover required to support his hypothesis presented itself after a 'natural experiment'. After recruitment of a new health officer in one of the districts, the rate of tonsillectomy in that school district dropped by a factor of ten within a year, and remained low for years afterwards. This sharp decline in rates was attributed to the difference in clinical judgement of the two physicians (Wennberg, 2010).

Studies of practice styles suggest that variations in clinical judgement could arise from clinician characteristics (age, sex, qualifications, and experience), clinician preferences, incentive mechanisms, availability of guidance, and the strength of evidence on effective treatments. The impact of clinician characteristics, incentives, and professional consensus on clinical decisions vary by setting. For example, high referral rates to secondary care by general practitioners in Norway were associated with the GPs' sex and specialist qualifications in family medicine (Ringberg et al., 2013). An earlier review of determinants of GP referral rates had concluded that less than 10 per cent of variation in referral rates could be explained by GP and practice characteristics, but highlighted intrinsic psychological variables, such as a GP's willingness to take risks, their tolerance of uncertainty or their perception of the frequency with which serious disease occurs, as important determinants of clinical decision-making (O'Donnell, 2000).

Research by John Wennberg showed that when there is strong evidence and a professional consensus that an intervention is effective, there tends to be little or no variation in clinical practice (such as hip fracture repair, colectomy for colorectal cancer). However, clinical practice variations are high for interventions where there is weak evidence of effectiveness and professional uncertainty (as for tonsillectomy, radical prostatectomy) (Wennberg, 2010). Figure 7.8 demonstrates the extent of variations for several common surgical procedures among Medicare patients for 306 referral regions in the USA.

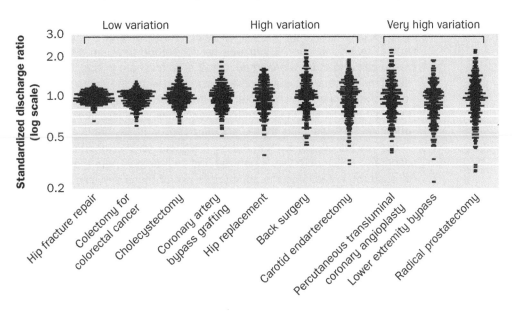

Figure 7.8 Rates of common surgical procedures among Medicare patients for 306 referral regions

Source: Reproduced from Mulley, A.G. (2009) Inconvenient truths about supplier induced demand and unwarranted variation in medical practice, *British Medical Journal*, 339: b4073, with permission from BMJ Publishing Group Ltd.

As previously discussed, availability of resources and clinical judgement are related, with many clinical decisions being influenced by the availability of particular services. This relationship was highlighted over 50 years ago by a public health researcher Milton Roemer, who stated: 'Hospital beds, once built, will be used' (Roemer, 1961). Increased bed availability is associated with an increase in admissions and in the USA, higher supply of health care resources overall is associated with more intense care, particularly for long-term illness (Wennberg, 2010).

Note that the main reason for *international variations* in utilization rates is the availability of services. In addition, morbidity rate, professional judgement, and illness behaviour have some influence. In contrast, *variations within a country* are likely to be due to professional judgement and the availability of services.

Unwarranted variation and categories of care

John Wennberg and colleagues argue that the causes of and the remedies for unwarranted variation differ according to three categories of care: effective care, preference-sensitive care, and supply-sensitive care (Trustees of Dartmouth College, 2016; Wennberg, 2010, 2011).

Effective care refers to services that are evidence-based in which the benefits clearly outweigh the risks. Variations in care for these services reflect failure to deliver needed care ('underuse'). Underuse of effective care is common, even in settings that are considered to be providing a high quality of care. There was no correlation between availability of resources and more widespread use of effective care in the USA. In fact, health care spending was inversely correlated with the likelihood of receiving recommended care: people who lived in higher spending regions or received care in hospitals with more resources were *less likely* to receive effective services than those receiving care in more deprived settings. These results suggested that the main reasons for the variations were the degree to which care was organized and coordinated, and the availability of systems to facilitate the appropriate use of these services for all eligible patients.

Preference-sensitive care is when more than one generally accepted treatment option is available, and where options have different risks and benefits and patients' attitudes towards those risks may vary. While the right rate should depend on patients' own values and informed patient choice, treatment rates can vary extensively because of differences in professional opinion. As discussed earlier, if the strength of evidence is poor for various treatment options, recommendations for treatments might be based on subjective opinion, personal experience, anecdote or an untested clinical theory. Patients also commonly delegate decision-making to physicians, under the assumption that they can accurately understand patients' values and recommend the correct treatment for them. This might not necessarily be true, as was seen in Hawker and colleagues' (2001) study of arthroplasty rates in Ontario, Canada. Wennberg argues that beyond the ongoing effort to reduce scientific uncertainty about the outcomes of various treatments, reducing unwarranted variation in preference-sensitive care could be through a shift in the doctor–patient relationship that reduces the influence of medical opinion and enhances the role of patient preferences through shared decision-making and informed patient choice.

Supply-sensitive care includes services for which the capacity of the local health care system (such as the supply of physicians and equipment) has a direct influence on utilization rates. Wennberg and colleagues (2002) observed that most of the variation in supply-sensitive care arises from the frequency with which patients with long-term diseases use consultations, diagnostic tests, referrals to medical specialists, hospitalizations, and stays in intensive care units. For each of these services, the per capita quantity of healthcare resources allocated to a given population largely determines the frequency of use. Both in the USA and England, the intensity of inpatient care, particularly for chronic conditions and terminal care, varies extensively across regions. In the USA, regions with high rates of use of supply-sensitive care do not have better overall outcomes as measured by mortality and indicators of the quality of care, suggesting that there is 'overuse' of these services. Reducing the overuse of supply-sensitive care requires organized systems of delivery that can manage care of a population of patients over time and across locations of care, and adjusting capacity to reflect medical evidence and patient preferences.

A summary of the factors that influence utilization, by categories of care, is provided in Table 7.1.

Table 7.1 Categories of medical services

Category of care	Factors that influence utilization			
	Medical theory	Medical evidence	Per capita supply of resources	Importance of patients' preferences
Effective care	Strong	Strong	Weak	Weak
Preference-sensitive care	Strong	Variable	Variable	Strong
Supply-sensitive care	Weak	Weak	Strong	Variable

Source: Wennberg et al. (2002). Copyrighted and published by Project HOPE/Health Affairs as Wennberg, J.E., Fisher, E.S. and Skinner, J.S., Geography And The Debate Over Medicare Reform, *Health Affairs (Millwood)* published online February 13, 2002; doi:10.1377/hlthaff.w2.96. Exhibit 1: Categories of Medical Services.

Activity 7.7

Based on your experience, provide examples from primary and hospital care of effective care, preference-sensitive care, and supply-sensitive care.

Feedback

Your responses will reflect your experience and setting.

1 Effective care:

- *Primary care* – immunizations for children, beta-blockers for heart attack patients or haemoglobin A1c testing for diabetic patients.
- *Secondary care* – surgery for hip fracture, angioplasty for heart attack.

2 Preference-sensitive care:

- *Primary care* – psychotherapy for mild psychological conditions, routine health checks for the elderly.
- *Hospital care* – elective surgery, hip and knee replacement for arthritis; caesarean section for singleton, non-breech deliveries; hysterectomy for abnormal uterine bleeding; mastectomy for early-stage breast cancer.

3 Supply-sensitive care:

- *Primary care* – physician visits, diagnostic tests.
- *Hospital care* – diagnostic procedures, hospital admissions for ambulatory care sensitive conditions when they can be managed in primary care.

Summary

In this chapter, you have read about a typology of health and health care needs. Felt need is determined by the individually perceived need for health. Depending on illness behaviour, felt need may be turned into an expressed need or demand for health care. Normative need depends on professional judgement about the capacity to benefit from care. Use of health services is strongly influenced by clinical judgement.

Use can be assessed by service-based and population-based measurements. Utilization rates vary internationally and within a country, depending on several demand and supply factors. The key question is whether use of services reflects health care needs. Analysis must take account of the socio-demographic factors affecting need and consider use/need ratios to analyse whether higher utilization rates reflect higher levels of need. Socio-economic status is an important determinant not only of morbidity and mortality but also of health care utilization. This fact requires careful consideration when planning and evaluating health services.

References

Ancona, C., Agabiti, N., Forastiere, F., Arca, M., Fusco, D., Ferro, S. et al. (2000) Coronary artery bypass graft surgery: socioeconomic inequalities in access and in 30 day mortality. A population-based study in Rome, Italy, *Journal of Epidemiology and Community Health*, 54 (12): 930–5.

Black, N.A., Langham, S. and Petticrew, M. (1995) Coronary revascularisation: why do rates vary geographically in the UK?, *Journal of Epidemiology and Community Health*, 49 (4): 408–12.

Collinson, P. (2010) British dentistry is in a painful state, *The Guardian*, 26 June 2010. Available at: http://www.theguardian.com/money/blog/2010/jun/26/dentists-health-and-wellbeing (accessed 19 April 2016).

Dixon, A., Le Grand, J., Henderson, J., Murray, R. and Poteliakhoff, E. (2007) Is the British National Health Service equitable? The evidence on socioeconomic differences in utilization, *Journal of Health Services Research and Policy*, 12 (2): 104–9.

Donohue, J.M., Morden, N.E., Gellad, W.F., Bynum, J.P., Zhou, W., Hanlon, J.T. et al. (2012) Sources of regional variation in Medicare: Part D drug spending, *New England Journal of Medicine*, 366 (6): 530–8.

Glover, A.J. (1938) The incidence of tonsillectomy in school children, *Proceedings of the Royal Society of Medicine*, 31 (10): 1219–36.

Hart, J.T. (1971) The inverse care law, *Lancet*, 1 (7696): 405–12.

Hawker, G.A., Wright, J.G., Coyte, P.C., Williams, J.I., Harvey, B., Glazier, R. et al. (2001) Determining the need for hip and knee arthroplasty: the role of clinical severity and patients' preferences, *Medical Care*, 39 (3): 206–16.

Last, J.L. (1963) The iceberg: completing the clinical picture in general practice, *Lancet*, ii: 28–31.

Le Grand, J. (1978) The distribution of public expenditure and the case of health care, *Economica*, 45 (178): 125–42.

Mackenbach, J.P., Slobbe, L., Looman, C.W.N., ven der Heide, A., Polder, J. and Garssen, J. (2011) Sharp upturn of life expectancy in the Netherlands: effect of more health care for the elderly?, *European Journal of Epidemiology*, 26 (12): 903–14.

Mackenbach, J.P., Stirbu, I., Roskam, A.J., Schaap, M.M., Menvielle, G., Leinsalu, M. et al. (2008) Socioeconomic inequalities in health in 22 European countries, *New England Journal of Medicine*, 358 (23): 2468–81.

Mulley, A.G. (2009) Inconvenient truths about supplier induced demand and unwarranted variation in medical practice, *British Medical Journal*, 339: b4073.

Neuburger, J., Hutchings, A., Allwood, D., Black, N. and van der Meulen, J.H. (2012) Sociodemographic differences in the severity and duration of disease amongst patients undergoing hip or knee replacement surgery, *Journal of Public Health (Oxford)*, 34 (3): 421–9.

NHS England, Public Health England and NHS Right Care (2015) *The NHS Atlas of Variation in Healthcare: Reducing unwarranted variation to increase value and improve quality*. Available at: http://www.rightcare.nhs.uk/index.php/atlas/nhs-atlas-of-variation-in-healthcare-2015/ (accessed 19 April 2016).

O'Donnell, C.A. (2000) Variation in GP referral rates: what can we learn from the literature?, *Family Practice*, 17 (6): 462–71.

Organization for Economic Cooperation and Development (OECD) (2014) *Geographic Variations in Health Care: What do we know and what can be done to improve health system performance?*, OECD Health Policy Studies Series. Paris: OECD Publishing.

Palència, L., Espelt, A., Rodríguez-Sanz, M., Rocha, K.B., Pasarín, M.I. and Borrell, C. (2013) Trends in social class inequalities in the use of health care services within the Spanish National Health System, 1993–2006. *European Journal of Health Economics*, 14 (2): 211–19.

Polikowski, M. and Santos-Eggimann, B. (2002) How comprehensive are the basic packages of health services? An international comparison of six health insurance systems, *Journal of Health Services Research and Policy*, 7 (3): 133–42.

Ringberg, U., Fleten, N., Deraas, T.S., Hasvold, T. and Förde, O.H. (2013). High referral rates to secondary care by general practitioners in Norway are associated with GPs' gender and specialist qualifications in family medicine: a study of 4350 consultations, *BMC Health Services Research*, 23 (13): 147.

Roemer, M.I. (1961) Bed supply and hospital utilization: a natural experiment, *Hospitals*, 1 (35): 36–42.

Stevens, A. and Gabbay, J. (1991) Needs assessment needs assessment . . . , *Health Trends*, 23: 20–3.

Sullivan, C.O., Omar R.Z., Ambler, G. and Majeed, A. (2005) Case-mix and variation in specialist referrals in general practice, *British Journal of General Practice*, 55 (516): 529–33.

Trustees of Dartmouth College (2016) *The Dartmouth Atlas of Health Care: Key issues*. Available at: http://www.dartmouthatlas.org/keyissues/.

van Doorslaer, E., Masseria, C., Koolman, X., and for the OECD Health Equity Research Group (2006) Inequalities in access to medical care by income in developed countries, *Canadian Medical Association Journal*, 174 (2): 177–83.

Vehvilainen, A.T., Kumpusalo, E.A, Voutilainen, S.O. and Takala, J.K. (1996) Does the doctors' professional experience reduce referral rates? Evidence from the Finnish referral study, *Scandinavian Journal of Primary Health Care*, 14 (1): 13–20.

Wennberg, J.E. (2010) *Tracking Medicine: A researcher's quest to understand health care*. New York: Oxford University Press.

Wennberg, J.E. (2011) Time to tackle unwarranted variations in practice, *British Medical Journal*, 342: d1513.

Wennberg, J.E., Fisher, E.S. and Skinner, J.S. (2002) Geography and the debate over Medicare reform, *Health Affairs (Millwood)* (suppl. web exclusive), February: W96–114. Available at: http://content.healthaffairs.org/content/early/2002/02/13/hlthaff.w2.96.full.pdf+html.

World Bank (2015) *World Development Indicators 2015*. Available at: http://data.worldbank.org/data-catalog/world-development-indicators.

World Health Organization/United Nations International Children's Emergency Fund (WHO/UNICEF) (2015) *Global Immunisation Data Coverage Estimates*, 2014 revision, July 2015. Available at: http://www.who.int/immunization/monitoring_surveillance/data/en/ (accessed 19 April 2016).

Ye, J., Zhang, J., Mikolajczyk, R., Torloni, M.R., Gülmezoglu, A.M. and Betran, A.P. (2016) Association between rates of caesarean section and maternal and neonatal mortality in the 21st century: a worldwide population-based ecological study with longitudinal data, *BJOG: An International Journal of Obstetrics and Gynaecology*, 123 (5): 745–53.

Users of health care   8

In this chapter, you will look at the various roles played by users of health services. You will explore how context influences the relationship between users and health services, and how the different roles of users impact on their involvement in health care. In exploring these roles, you will look at the interpersonal relationships between patients and health care staff and the psychosocial factors affecting the process of communication. You will look at the interactions of users in their roles as consumers, citizens, and as members of communities. You will consider the potential roles that citizens might play in policy-making, including who should be consulted. Finally, you will look at the different ways that communities have been included.

Learning objectives

After working through this chapter, you will be able to:

- outline factors that influence the style of staff–patient interaction
- suggest reasons for failure to communicate with patients
- give examples of how to improve the staff–patient relationship
- outline the concept of consumerism in health services
- outline the role of context in shaping the relationship between provider and users of services
- give examples of initiatives to strengthen consumer power and community participation in health care
- discuss the ways in which the public can be involved in health care policy-making

Key terms

Bureaucracy: A formal type of organization involving hierarchy, impersonality, continuity, and expertise.

Community participation: A process by which individuals or groups assume responsibility for health matters of their community.

Compliance: The extent to which a patient follows professional advice.

Consumerism: A social movement promoting and representing user interests in health services.

Empathy: A response that demonstrates understanding and acceptance of the patient's feelings and concerns.

Encounter: The interaction of two or more people in a face-to-face meeting.

Social role: A set of ideas and actions that let individuals behave according to expected social norms.

Users of health care – as patients, consumers, communities, and citizens

In Chapter 5, you explored power as a key concept in understanding professionalism and identified the attributes of professional power. One aspect of this is the relative power of users of services. In this chapter, you will explore the different roles that users take within health services and how these roles reflect different degrees of power. The model of health care delivery will have an influence on these roles:

1 In a *professional model* of health care delivery, users are seen as patients. In this sense, you can think of patients as people expressing a felt need for better health in an *interpersonal* relationship with a health care worker, such as a doctor or nurse.
2 In a *market-driven model* of health care delivery, users are seen as consumers of health services. As consumers, people are aware of their knowledge, and make choices and influence the distribution and use of power. In this case, you can think of informed people selecting providers and insurance companies in competitive health care markets. In the consumerist view, users are seen as *customers* of health services.
3 In the *community model*, users are the 'public' participating in health care issues. The public in this case may have multiple faces. These may be self-defined groups sharing something in common and recognizing a collective experience (for example, local residents, the diabetic community), as well as the wider public as taxpayers. In the community model, users are seen as *citizens* taking an active role in health services.

In the following sections, you will examine these different roles, beginning with the role of users as patients, and the important relationship between the patient and health care professional.

Users as patients

Why study staff–patient interaction?

Much of the research, at least in high-income countries, has focused on the interaction between staff and patients. There are many reasons why staff–patient interactions are an important concern for practitioners and managers. In the first instance, poor communication between staff and patients is a major reason for dissatisfaction and a poor outcome of care.

Research in the UK in the early 1990s illustrates the importance of communication in patients' experiences with general practitioners. In one study, 27 per cent of patients were critical of the treatment they received. However, of these, 27 per cent criticized the practitioner for their lack of responsiveness and cooperation, and a further 25 per cent criticized the personal attributes of the health professional. Only 4 per cent of respondents criticized mistakes made by the practitioner. The authors concluded that the doctor's 'ability to dispense pills is not in question but his manner – abrupt and abrasive – calls into question his ability as a general practitioner' (Nettleton and Harding, 1994). These findings are consistent with those of a previous study, which reported patients' views of the relative importance of different attributes. Most important was that the doctor provided sufficient information; second, that the doctor was 'likeable'; third, that the consultation was long enough; and fourth, that the doctor had good medical skills (Williams and Calnan, 1991).

The impact of communication between health staff and patients on outcomes of care is well documented. For example, instruction and encouragement of patients can reduce post-operative pain (Egbert et al., 1964). Patients who received extra visits from anaesthetists were able to leave hospital three days earlier than those who did not.

In the USA, studies of the high frequency of litigation suggest that failure to communicate adequately with patients is a significant reason for patients to take action (Levinson et al., 1997). The failure to communicate with patients is related to three areas:

1 *Failure to assess the full spectrum of patient concerns.* In a study of routine encounters, patients were typically interrupted after 18 seconds.
2 *Failure to develop and maintain therapeutic relations.* Failure to develop empathy, a response demonstrating an accurate understanding and acceptance of a patient's feelings. Developing empathy reduces negative emotions such as anger, anxiety, and depression, which are common reactions to illness.
3 *Failure to deliver information to patients.* Levels of distress are reduced when patients perceive themselves to have received adequate information on diagnostic procedures and treatment plans. The most challenging aspect for staff is communicating bad news to patients and their families.

Factors influencing the staff–patient encounter

Many factors are known to influence staff–patient encounters. These include:

- patient's socio-economic status
- severity of disease
- type of setting (home care/institutional care)
- patient's knowledge
- method of paying for care.

The following activity will provide you with an opportunity to explore some factors in staff–patient interactions.

✎ Activity 8.1

Poor interaction between practitioners and patients, leading to patient dissatisfaction, is a common problem in many contexts. The following article by Michael Bernhart and colleagues describes a study undertaken in Indonesia in 1998, which tried to overcome people's reluctance to criticize health services. As you read the article, consider the following:

1 How did the researchers try and achieve this?
2 How successful were they?
3 What were the principal sources of dissatisfaction?

Patient satisfaction in developing countries

There have been several efforts to elicit constructive criticism from clients of Indonesian health care facilities but the responses from clients have been uniformly laudatory. As examples: a survey of 4000 patients of a primary care facility in Jakarta found that 94.7% of the respondents were fully satisfied. A similar survey of 1200 patients in three health centers conducted by the East Java Province Health Office found the satisfaction rate at 93.2% ... They are almost certainly not representative of true feelings given that drop-out rates from preventive and chronic curative services range from 25 to 35% and less than one in four citizens uses the public sector primary care facilities. More intensive grilling of patients does not seem to change the result; a similar finding was produced in a study of women in West Java using antenatal care services which solicited opinions on 12 areas of client satisfaction (Sinyor, 1997). The interviewing was intensive (average duration of interview was 78 min); yet no respondent answered that she was dissatisfied with a single aspect of the services (5.3% did voice only moderate satisfaction with a few items). Again, the drop-out rate belies the rosy image projected by the results.

Research questions

If Indonesian patients normally withhold negative opinions or evaluative comments, would they be more forthcoming with factual information, even though that too might be interpreted negatively? The study reported in this paper addresses that question. The practical relevance of the question is that useful information on patient satisfaction might be obtained if clients are asked about events and behaviors, rather than for their opinions.

. . . A second challenge, not specific to Indonesia, is to identify those aspects of the service that are meaningful to patient satisfaction. Although a number of patient satisfaction studies have been conducted in Indonesia, it does not appear that any of them methodically determined the relevance to patients of the variables employed . . .

Method

A list of 14 factors thought to be potentially relevant to patient satisfaction was compiled. These factors came from examination of literature reviews on patient satisfaction and a series of focus groups conducted by Rusmiyati (1997) in West Java. These factors were framed in terms of events and observable behaviors, not opinions. To illustrate, patients were not asked whether they felt acceptable norms of privacy were observed, but rather they were asked whether anyone was present during examination, counseling and treatment who did not participate in providing care . . . Two of the 25 questions did elicit opinions: facility cleanliness, where the researchers could not agree on an objective indicator; and speed of service. The latter was to check perceptions of the wait against actual recorded time spent in the clinic.

Seventy-five patients were interviewed in 11 clinics on three islands. The islands were chosen to sample the breadth of diversity of Indonesia . . .

Results

Table [8.1] summarizes the findings on relative importance and the frequency of expressed negative information.

Frequency of critical or negative information

It may be observed from the right-hand column that negative responses were forthcoming from patients in far greater percentages than had been obtained in earlier opinion-based research. As examples of the constructive criticism offered, 28% of the respondents answered that someone not

Table 8.1 Relative importance of patient satisfaction factors and
frequency of negative responses

Patient satisfaction area	Importance score	Negative responses
To be cured	0.89	23%
Receive medicine	0.78	4
Privacy during examination	0.58	28
Cleanliness of the facility	0.57	65
Receiving full information on the name, nature, prognosis, management, and danger signs	0.55	38
Receiving intelligible answers to questions	0.53	20
Receiving encouragement to ask questions	0.52	75
Use of the household/indigenous language	0.44	11
Continuity of provider	0.41	51
Waiting time for service and total wait	0.40	14.31 min
Availability of a toilet	0.33	0
Cost of the service	0.31	1
Availability of a seat	0.30	1
Health worker engaging patient in social conversation	0.27	73

Source: Bernhart et al. (1999).

participating in their health care service had been present during the
examination. 38% had not received information and 65% faulted the
cleanliness of the facility . . .

Relative importance

The center column reports the relative ratings of importance; the range is
from 0 (least important) to 1.0 (most important). With rare exceptions
(eight of the 75 respondents) patients ranked being cured as the most
important aspect of the service. This was hardly unexpected, but its first
place finish provided reassurance that the answers on relative importance
were not given without thought. Patients ranked receiving medicine as
second most important and privacy as the third. There were further questions regarding privacy for women who were required to disrobe for the
examination. Against expectations, privacy was nearly as important an
aspect of care for men as for women.

As may be seen in Table [8.1] the top ranked issues were associated
with medical aspects of care (cure and medicine), followed, loosely, by
issues concerning personal dignity and completeness and intelligibility of

*counseling. Surprisingly, 'obvious' satisfaction issues such as cost, conti-
nuity, waiting time and amenities were relegated to the bottom of the list.
However, the low cost of service, built-in continuity of provider in the
smaller facilities and widespread availability of amenities may have
diminished patient concern with these factors.*

Consistency of responses among respondents

*As noted earlier, given the heterogeneity of the society, there was con-
cern that respondents of different cultural backgrounds would assign
different relative importance to the factors. It appears that they did not.
The consistency of response was assessed across regions, sexes and
purpose of visit to the facility; only the last produced variation.*

*There was no statistically detectable difference among relative rankings
of importance by region . . .*

Discussion

*. . . The assertion that patients were willing to provide critical information
should, perhaps, be rephrased to read that they will provide more critical
information. Although the politeness bias seems to give way when factual
information, not opinions, are requested, we cannot determine whether
the responses are fully candid. It was possible, however, to test the plausibility of some of the answers given. The five questions on counseling were
all followed by a request to the patient to describe the information given;
their answers were recorded and later rated for plausibility by an individual who did not collect the data. This is a slippery concept, to be sure, but
the research was not concerned with the accuracy of the counseling
given – simply whether counseling was provided as claimed by the patient –
and the patients' answers were scored as 'plausible' if the content of their
answer was something a health worker could have plausibly said.*

Reprinted from Bernhart, M., Wiadyana, I.G.P., Wihardjo, H., Pohan, I. (1999) Patient
satisfaction in developing countries, *Social Science & Medicine*, 48:989–96, with permission from Elsevier.

Feedback

1 People were asked about events and behaviours, rather than for their
   opinions. It was hoped that if patients asked for information that
   might be verified, they would be more likely to answer based on their
   experience in the clinic.
2 Negative responses were forthcoming from patients in far greater
   percentages than had been obtained in earlier opinion-based research.
3 Not encouraged to ask questions (75 per cent); health worker did not
   engage patient in social conversation (73 per cent); facility not clean
   (65 per cent); and lack of continuity of provider (51 per cent).

Compliance and staff–patient interaction

Compliance (in the current context of health services) has been defined as the extent to which patients follow professional advice. Although socio-economic and cultural factors play an important role, staff–patient interaction also influences compliance with treatment (Sbaro and Sbaro, 1994). As an example, it is useful to look at tuberculosis (TB) control. Although a short-term combination chemotherapy is effective and inexpensive, TB is still a major cause of death worldwide, killing 1.5 million people in 2013 (WHO, 2015). Notwithstanding the logistical difficulties of case detection in low-income countries, failure of compliance with treatment is considered a global problem. A high proportion of patients discontinue medication when they feel better, but are still infectious, and communicate the disease. Hopes are directed towards the development of even shorter treatment regimes, but effective interaction of health workers with patients forms a central part of any control strategy. In a number of low-income countries, the use of specially trained village health workers has proved successful in achieving high rates of case detection and compliance. A study of this approach in Bangladesh attributed the success to the trust that these workers enjoy within the local communities (Chowdhury et al., 1997).

Societal forces shaping the staff–patient encounter

So far, you have looked at the difficulties of the staff–patient encounter. But what are the forces underlying this relationship? What makes patients and staff act as they do?

Sociological research has identified some general principles underlying the staff–patient interaction. Cross-cultural research suggests that these can be found in all cultures. It is clear that relative power and routine work are important concepts explaining the position of patients. In this section, you will look at these two concepts and some attributes that influence the relationship between staff and patients in a little more detail:

1 *Relative power*: Patients are in a weak bargaining position. They are vulnerable and helpless, and many are ill informed about their status. The experience of illness leads them to seek a passive role. However, this situation is changing in countries, as patients gain confidence and acquire knowledge about their condition (see below).
2 *Routine work*: Patients are treated as objects of work and each client is one of many. What a patient perceives as a unique situation is routine for the staff.

Two factors that influence the staff–patient relationship are *cultural norms* and *bureaucracy*.

Cultural norms

Talcott Parsons (1902–1979) was one of the earliest sociologists to investigate the relationship between doctors and patients. Both doctors and patients are regarded as occupying *social roles*, which facilitate their interaction and define the expected behaviour of each.

Parsons is associated with the *functionalist* perspective (Parsons and Mayhew, 1982). Society is seen as a system in which each element serves a purpose or maintains a function; members of society fulfil their *roles* to meet society's needs because they share common goals and values. The role an individual occupies is related to social status, and represents a set of ideas and actions. Social functioning is achieved by individuals acting according to their expected role. For example, the *sick role* ensures social functioning by expecting people to behave according to social norms: unlike other forms of absenteeism, sick leave is socially accepted. But employees are expected to return to work as soon as possible, as sick leave rates that are too high would impair economic performance.

You may also remember from previous chapters the functionalist view on women's role in lay care and on the role of doctors as professionals. Although the functionalist perspective was influential in the 1950s, it has been criticized for taking too little account of change and conflict in society.

In Parsons' view, both roles – that of the patient (the 'sick' role) and that of the doctor – involve *privileges* and *obligations*. Table 8.2 outlines the *privileges* and *obligations* of the two roles (Parsons, 1951).

Note that this model describes an ideal interaction between doctor and patient. The model has been criticized for its basis in one-off interactions that do not represent the majority of health care encounters. Importantly, the model does not apply to chronic disease, as this relies on multiple interactions over time and requires a much more complex pattern of care

Table 8.2 Parsons' doctor and patient privileges and obligations

	Privileges	Obligations
Patient ('sick role')	The right to be exempted from normal activity (for example, not going to work) Being regarded as in need of care and not being blamed for own illness.	To seek medical advice To want to get well as quickly as possible
Doctor	To examine patients physically and psychologically Afforded professional autonomy and authority	To be objective and neutral (for example, not to judge patients' behaviour on moral grounds) To use professional skills for the welfare of patients and the community (rather than for self-interest).

and constant adaptation to the changing nature of the illness. Mol (2008) captures the complexity of chronic care in her book *The Logic of Care*, including the increasing role that patients play in monitoring their own health, and adjusting their care accordingly, outside their interaction with the doctor. An example is the role that the diabetic patient takes in monitoring blood glucose levels and 'fine-tuning' insulin intakes accordingly. Parsons' functionalist view has also been criticized for its affirmation of the doctor's control function and for assuming a lack of conflict between the roles of patients and doctors.

The patient's right to stay off work is an important constituent of the sick role. Obviously, how it works varies with social and cultural context. On average, sick leave is shorter in Japan and America than in Europe. Within countries, it is shorter in the private sector than the public sector. Role performance depends also on economic factors. Time off work by the workforce is higher during economic growth and lower in periods of recession and job insecurity.

Bureaucracy

Bureaucracy is a common phenomenon of large organizations, including health services. In Weber's view, bureaucratic organization is a consequence of increasing complexity in the division of labour (Weber, 1922). Most people have come across the negative sides of bureaucracy, such as the procedures that need to be followed to get anything done. To understand how bureaucracy affects communication with patients, you will need to understand its main properties. We now look at these properties in a little more detail:

1 *Hierarchy*: People engage in narrowly defined tasks and work under rules. Power is distributed according to defined areas of competence. Authority and responsibility are clearly defined for each member of staff. In the case of health services, doctors, nurses, and other health workers work in hierarchies with a number of different occupational roles oriented to different tasks.
2 *Continuity*: The system is self-sustaining. Written records ensure machine-like accuracy, even if staff change. For example, shifts are not supposed to affect patient care.
3 *Impersonality*: Work is done according to strict rules, without favouritism; officials are exchangeable. It gives officials the authority to act on behalf of the whole organization. For example, staff provide care according to agreed regimens and protocols.
4 *Expertise*: Officials are selected according to merit and are trained to have the necessary skills and knowledge to fulfil their function. You have seen how both doctors and nurses have designated training programmes with strict registration requirements, including continuing professional development.

All this contributes to a rational organization of labour but it also affects the interaction with patients, which can have negative implications. For example:

- the bureaucratic separation of tasks can result in fragmented care;
- patients may receive contradictory signals from different encounters;
- staff may develop stereotypical and unhelpful views of patients, judging their personality through the amount of work they cause.

Often, it is possible to observe an inverse relation between patient openness and position in the hierarchy: patients tend to talk more easily and more frankly to members of staff who occupy a lower position in the hierarchy, rather than to senior doctors and nurses.

The bureaucratic type of organization provides privileged social status and relative job security. It is often seen as the only means of providing services of equal standard throughout the country. However, as we have seen in previous chapters, other factors can influence the standard of services provided.

Contemporary changes in the patient role

In many countries, the role of the patient is changing in several ways; ways that one British commentator, Angela Coulter, has described:

> No longer is he or she simply a passive victim of illness. In the 21st century the patient is a decision-maker, care manager and co-producer of health, an evaluator, a potential change agent, a taxpayer and an active citizen whose voice must be heard by decision-makers. Acknowledging these roles and developing and extending active partnerships with patients has become essential for all health care providers, and in particular for those working on the front-line in primary care.

> The key to restoring confidence lies as much in the hands of clinicians as it does in politicians. Clinicians could do a great deal to help inform and educate those who seek their help. If the public can be helped to understand the limits of medical care as well as its potential benefits, they are much more likely to use health services appropriately and responsibly. Recognition of the patient as an active, autonomous player in the health care system should have profound consequences for the way in which health care is delivered. Relationships between health professionals and the public they serve need to be transformed at all levels, organizational as well as individual . . . Managers and clinicians will have to be prepared to cede some power and patients must be willing to take greater responsibility for their own health. These changes are necessary to ensure the sustainability of collective health care provision. (Coulter, 2002)

One example of users as 'co-producers of health' mentioned by Coulter (2002) is the increasing emphasis on *patient-centred care*. This model puts the patient's wishes at the centre of discussion (Berwick, 2009). Compliance in this model is viewed as ensuring that the intervention fits with the patient's life-style or condition (Aronson, 2007).

The model emphasizes the need for communication with the patient as well as involvement of the patient in their own care. The rise of chronic conditions has seen an increasing move to involve patients in their own care, providing them with the know-how and skills to expertly manage their condition (Lorig et al., 1999). In the UK, the Expert Patients Programme has provided training on ways to use medication, nutrition, as well as the proper use of the health system. In this approach, both patient and health professional bring their respective knowledge and skills to the interaction (Donaldson, 2003).

In the next sections, you will look at the other roles highlighted by Coulter (2002).

Users as consumers

The second model views users of health services as consumers, based on a consumerist view of health care.

The underlying view of consumerism is that providers tend to disregard consumer interests and therefore their rights need to be protected. Thus, provider power needs to be balanced by consumers who actively monitor and evaluate health services and who make informed choices.

In turn, giving people choice, for example, choice of provider, is thought to improve the quality of services and people's satisfaction. Consumer power is also seen to improve the responsiveness to complaints and strengthen people's rights. Health care is regarded like any other service, as a commodity that can be produced and consumed. However, there are a number of things that make health care different from other services. The following activity will help you think through why this is so.

Activity 8.2

Think about the following two situations – the first an interaction between a nurse and patient, and the second an interaction between a seller and buyer of a car. Now compare the consumer power in both cases. Note down the similarities and differences, and then compare your thoughts with the feedback below.

Feedback

The power of a car buyer depends on information. The key mechanism of consumer power is choice. If provided with the necessary information on the car market, consumers can choose between several models and car dealers. But the buyer may not have information as complete as that of the seller, an advantage that might be exploited.

In health care, consumer sovereignty is reduced due to uncertainty about the type and amount of care needed. Health care workers act as *agents*, deciding on behalf of people the type and amount of care that is to be consumed. In many contexts, health care is usually paid for indirectly through insurance contributions or taxation, unlike the car deal where money is paid for at the point of sale. In addition in health care, those who pay may be different from those who consume it.

In fact, consumerism appears to be the vehicle for different political interests (Lupton, 1997). Over the years, the discourse on consumerism has been adopted both by community groups focusing on patient autonomy, and by policy-makers who favour a free market model of health care. Therefore, it is important to be cautious and mindful of the different motives of the actors advocating consumerism.

Choice and community empowerment

As you have seen, the similarities between health care and consumption of commercial goods are limited. However, increasingly there is choice in logistical matters (e.g. choice of doctors and hospitals), in clinical matters (e.g. deciding between treatment alternatives), and in political matters (e.g. local participation in decision-making).

The extent of choice varies widely. In a number of countries, health care systems have responded to political demands and introduced various forms of public participation. Important, too, is defining and implementing people's rights. Political participation is part of a larger concept of community empowerment, a topic addressed in more detail below (Saltman, 1994).

Before that, however, it is important to consider the different degrees of power available to patients. One framework, the ladder of participation (Arnstein, 1969), describes the spectrum of possibilities, ranging from the traditional position in which the patient displays little power and is largely 'manipulated' by the health care professional through to the case where the patient takes control (see Figure 8.1).

Initiatives to strengthen consumer power

A number of initiatives have strengthened consumer power in health services (Saltman and Figueras, 1997). These revolve around better information,

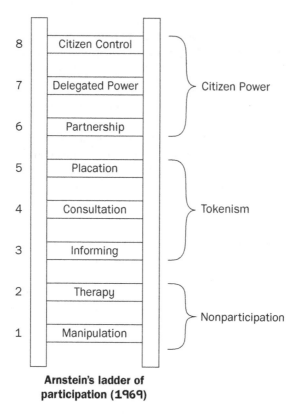

**Arnstein's ladder of
participation (1969)**

Figure 8.1 Ladder of participation
Source: Arnstein (1969).

systems to handle complaints, the representation of consumers at various levels of health services, and mechanisms to protect patients' rights.

The latter initiative has been approached in two main ways: charters setting out entitlements and expectations, and laws. The former is the approach adopted in the UK, where health care providers have developed explicit standards that patients can expect to receive. In contrast to a charter, other countries have defined patients' rights through law. Finland introduced legislation in 1993 that gives the patients' ombudsman an important role in monitoring and implementing all matters concerning patient rights. The Netherlands has introduced legally defined patient rights and enhanced the provisions to enforce those rights through courts. There is also formalized participation of consumers in the decision-making process of health care. In India, the government extended the Consumer Protection Act to private health services to ensure that patients receive appropriate quality of care. The objective was to provide a less costly remedy to consumer complaints than the more expensive civil litigation (Bhat, 1996).

There is no doubt that consumerism has been influential in challenging health care professions and increasing users' powers. But have these political processes also changed the health care encounter? You might expect that the patient in a role as consumer would reject paternalism and professional dominance, and actively assess – and, if necessary, counter – expert knowledge. Obviously, the encounter is more complex. Deborah Lupton, an Australian sociologist, has pointed out that seeing patients as consumers underestimates the cultural and emotional features that influence the staff–patient relationship. The feeling of dependency is central to the illness experience and may work against taking up a consumerist position. Illness, pain, and disability tend to encourage a need for trust in experts and faith in health care. From her research in Australia, there is evidence that the role patients take depends on their personal circumstances. In the health care encounter, patients may both pursue the ideal type 'active consumer' or 'passive patient' position, simultaneously or variously, depending on the context (Lupton, 1997). As we discussed earlier in the chapter, the role of the patient is changing, at least in some countries.

Users as communities and citizens

The other key roles highlighted by Coulter (2002) at the beginning of this chapter include users as taxpayers and citizens. There is growing recognition that the responsibility for health is distributed within society and that there is a role for the user as a citizen with responsibilities as well as rights. This has led to increasing attempts to involve users in the planning of health services and in developing policy.

There are several proposed benefits to this, including enhancing public accountability as well as addressing 'the democratic deficit'. In addition, this approach is seen as helping to meet the expectations of an increasingly knowledgeable public (Cooper et al., 1995).

Activity 8.3

The following edited extract from an article by Jonathan Lomas (1997), a Canadian health services researcher, focuses on the types of decision for which there is a potential role for public input into publicly funded health services. As you read it, consider the author's attitude to the following:

1 The reason why formal carers and policy-makers are interested in lay involvement.
2 The reasons why policy-makers need to be cautious in their expectations of lay involvement in the three key areas of decisions about funding, service provision, and rationing.

Reluctant rationers: public input to health care priorities

Collective health care decisions and public input

It is no coincidence that public interest in public involvement in health care decisions has occurred at the same time as concern about the ability of the state to continue to fund ever higher levels of service. Health care system providers and managers, as well as their public funders, are faced with increasingly tough and painful choices in the allocation of resources within and/or to the health care system. Not surprisingly, they are looking to share some of this pain with the public. The desire of governments, managers and providers for public input is, therefore, largely instrumental; they do not see public involvement as a goal in itself. These decision-makers wish to find ways to have the public take (or at least share) ownership of the tough choices they face in allocating increasingly scarce resources . . .

From this perspective, there are certain expectations of public involvement: first, that representative individuals are willing and feel able to be involved – unwilling participants are unlikely to take or share ownership in the eventual decisions; second, that the public accepts the need to ration within a fixed public budget for health care – the alternative merely posits more resources as the solution; third, that mechanisms are available to ensure that public input generates representative views – this not being the case, a false 'public' imprimatur is placed on the lobbying positions of over-represented interests such as particular disease groups or health care employees; fourth, the public will not override unambiguous information on the ineffectiveness of various service options – ignoring such data leads to less 'health' being produced for the same funds; and finally, that members of the public are willing and able to adopt a collective view rather than a self-interested view – allocation of public resources for health care is more about what communities need than about what individuals want . . .

Defining essential or core services, prioritization, or rationing are three of the most common phrases used to describe the gradual transformation of implicit rules into explicit processes for resource allocation. Many countries have involved the public to some degree. The most publicized has been the Oregon process. Unfortunately, this exercise in democratic rationing provides few lessons about methodologies for collective decision-making (it was about the non-poor allocating health care resources for the poor), or those considering the breadth of possible public input to health care decisions (it addressed only public input to specific services that should be offered).

Table [8.3] outlines six questions under three types of collective decision-making for which there is a potential role for the public . . . The majority of reported exercises have tended to start out with a primary focus on

Table 8.3 Six collective health care decisions for which there is a potential role for public input

Type of decision	Specific question	Role
Service funding	1. *Funding level*: what should be the level of public funding for the provision of health care services?	Taxpayer
	2. *Funding arrangements*: under what financing and organizational arrangements should services be offered?	
Services to offer	3. *Broad service categories*: what broad categories of service should be offered as part of the publicly funded health care system?	Collective decision-maker
	4. *Specific services*: what specific services should be offered within each broad category of publicly funded health care?	
Who should receive services?	5. *Clinical circumstances*: what are the clinical circumstances of patients who should receive specific offered services?	Patient perspective
	6. *Socio-demographic circumstances*: what are the socio-demographic circumstances of patients who should receive specific offered services?	

Source: Lomas (1997).

question 4, motivated by the apparent need to limit the service package available to the public within a jurisdiction. The complexity of the task has, however, driven most of these exercises back to question 3 – 'What broad categories of service should be offered . . .?'

The purpose of Table [8.3] is not, however, just to point out the limited nature of current exercises. Rather, it is to show that not only do individuals think as three persons within one – taxpayer with views about funding, collective decision-maker with opinions about services offered and patient with preferences about services received – but also that the system would require him or her to think in three different ways if he or she were to contribute comprehensively to health care decision-making.

Decisions on public funding

. . . As taxpayers, individuals appear to support increased funding for health care, at the expense of almost all other areas of public expenditure . . . From governments' current perspective of expenditure reductions, public input on the level of funding for health care may, therefore, be best left unsought.

. . . Our own research in Canada found that the average citizen was not interested in being involved in these funding decisions . . . These were decisions deemed appropriate for politicians and the experts. Furthermore,

*few individuals are interested in how the state chooses to pay its provid-
ers or organize the system; they are principally concerned about getting
to see a provider when they want one.*

Decisions on what services to offer under public funding

*The second category of decision-making – what services to offer – is
where public input to priority-setting has focused most. The limits on public funding are, in this case, achieved by rationing services. Although
many exercises have failed to make it explicit, the presumed role for individuals is as collective decision-makers, i.e. to decide not what services
they personally wish to see offered but rather what services they believe
would best serve the general community good. The overall level and
arrangement of funding, whether decided via public input or not, are obviously the constraining influences.*

*If the task of priority-setting is done at the level of broad service categories,
such as 'nursing care', 'services for acute emergencies', 'preventive care'
and so on, it appears that the public are at least able to provide reasonably consistent relative priorities. This approach was reflected in the 1994
World Bank Report with the recommendation that public funding should
be reserved for essential services, defined with community input, and
oriented in developing countries towards 'primary care'.*

*Average citizens are, however, largely reticent about their ability to per-
form this collective decision-maker role . . . in Canada two-thirds of individuals did not want to take responsibility for priority-setting. Once the
collective decision-making turns to priorities amongst specific services
such as types of surgery, treatment for addictions, specific diagnostic
tests and so on, both the consistency of responses and the willingness of
individuals to participate decline even further . . .*

*This is hardly surprising given the information needs. Focusing on specific
services invites consideration of its costs and benefits in precise terms;
this is information that is often either not available or not readily understandable to the average citizen. The more specific the service over which
citizens are being asked to pass a priority judgement, then the more they
are driven to want to know its costs and benefits for specific clinical and
social circumstances. In the absence of such information, the public is
being asked to do the logically absurd task of judging need (and, hence,
priority) independently of patient circumstance . . .*

Decisions on who should receive offered services

*The third category of decisions is the specific circumstances of patients
who should receive particular services, once it has been established
that the services will be offered. In this case, restrictions on public funding relate to rationing among patients not services. Denying access to*

services offered under public funding whether because of clinical or socio-demographic characteristics of a patient, has become a contentious element of many health care systems, potentially resulting in legal challenge. The contentious and sharply distributive nature of these questions takes us into the realm of moral philosophy.

. . . Using practice guidelines, some jurisdictions have put much (probably misplaced) faith in this approach to limiting the growth of medical services. Although in some cases these clinical considerations can be relatively straightforward, more often than not the task is technically challenging and demanding of expertise. It is not clear that there is any substantial role for public input to these expert decisions.

This is probably not true, however, for the socio-demographic characteristics of patients which might limit access to offered services. Factors such as age and lifestyle have either been used or came under consideration for use as ways of excluding some patients from receiving publicly funded services . . . Interestingly, in explicit exercises members of the public appear to be more willing than physicians and managers to ration services on the basis of such socio-demographic characteristics.

. . . involvement of members of the public is politically advisable given the sensitive nature of decisions to deny patients access to services on the basis of their age, lifestyle or social circumstance. One would hope, however, that final decisions on such denials of access to services would not allow public views to over-ride existing protections for minorities, the disabled, or others, embodied within human rights legislation.

Reproduced from Lomas (1997). With permission of the Royal Society of Medicine Press Limited.

Feedback

1 To share some of the pain of making hard choices with the public.
2 As regards public involvement in funding decisions, they generally want to increase spending on health care despite governments' desire to control spending; for decisions as to what services to provide, the public often feel ill-equipped and reluctant to be involved; and the public find the task of rationing (at the level of individual patients) too technically challenging, though no such reluctance exists if the decisions are limited to socio-demographic factors such as age or sex.

An example of the latter comes from a survey carried out by Ann Bowling in the mid-1990s in which she sought the views of a large nationally representative sample of adults on priorities for health services (Bowling, 1996). An interview survey based on a random sample of people aged 16 and over in Great Britain was undertaken. The response rate to the survey was

75 per cent, and the total number of adults interviewed was 2005. Respondents were asked to prioritize twelve services. In addition, their attitudes to who should set priorities and allocate budgets were sought. The results showed that the highest priority was accorded to 'treatments for children with life-threatening illness'; the next highest priority was accorded to 'special care and pain relief for people who are dying'. The lowest priorities were given to 'treatment for infertility' and 'treatment for people aged 75 and over with life-threatening illness'. Most respondents thought that surveys like this one should be used in the planning of health services. Bowling concluded that the public prioritize treatments specifically for younger rather than older people and there is some public support for people with self-inflicted conditions (for example, through tobacco smoking) receiving lower priority for care.

Activity 8.4

Despite Lomas' concerns about the role of the public in making policy about which services should be provided, numerous attempts have been made to involve them in this way. A review of the published accounts of such efforts in the UK, the USA, Canada, Sweden, and Australia found little evidence that involving the public (limited to patients in this case) had led to improvements in the quality of health care (Crawford et al., 2002).

As you read the following extract from Crawford and colleagues' paper, note the three reasons the authors give to be cautious in interpreting these findings as discouraging.

Systematic review of involving patients in the planning and development of health care

A review of more than 300 papers on involving patients in the planning and development of health care found that . . . involving patients has contributed to changes to services. The effects of involvement on accessibility and acceptability of services or impact on the satisfaction, health, or quality of life of patients have not been examined . . . A potential problem in interpreting the results is that publication bias may favour the publication of reports from initiatives that were judged to be successful.

Several factors may account for our central finding, the limited amount of information about the effects of involving patients. The aims of involving patients have always been broader than just improving the quality of health care. Involving patients has been viewed by many as a democratic or ethical requirement: because patients pay for services, they have a right to influence how they are managed. An alternative view is that involving patients is not intended to devolve power to patients but to legitimize the decisions of policy makers and administrators. It is argued that through consulting with users of health services, support for decisions that would otherwise be unpopular can be obtained. Such aims imply that establishing mechanisms for involving patients should be seen as an end in itself rather than as a means of improving the quality of services. However, initiatives that fall short of bringing about changes to services are not in keeping with the aims of current policy or patients.

The effects of involving patients are likely to be complex, affecting different aspects of services in different ways. The views of patients are among many factors that influence change in health services, and providers of health care remain the final arbiter of how much weight is attached to patients' views. Separating out change specifically attributable to the participation of patients is a difficult task . . . Patients' involvement is not without its costs, and including outcome measures in future evaluations of involving patients could enable comparisons of different approaches and evaluation of the effects of suggestions made by patients.

. . . This absence of evidence should not be mistaken for an absence of effect. Health care providers may be increasingly required to demonstrate that they involve patients in the planning process, but they will also continue to be accountable for the decisions they make.

Reprinted from Crawford, M.J. et al. (2002) in *BMJ*, 325:1263–8, with permission from BMJ Publishing Group Ltd.

Feedback

The three reasons suggested are:

1 Improvement in health care is not the only objective of involving the public. Other worthy objectives are to be as democratic as possible and to gain public ownership of hard decisions. The achievement of these objectives should also be considered.
2 It is difficult to separate the effect of public involvement from other influences on decisions.
3 Absence of evidence is not the same as absence of effect.

Two British commentators, Dominique Florin and Jennifer Dixon (2004), have explained the potential benefits of greater public involvement.

Public involvement in health care services

Advocates of increased public involvement argue that public services are paid for by the people and therefore should be shaped more extensively by them, preferably by a fully representative sample. One assumption made is that greater public involvement will lead to more democratic decision making and, in turn, better accountability, but neither is necessarily the case. A second assumption is that more public involvement is an intrinsic good. This belief is based on values or ideology and thus cannot be tested, but it is often allied to beliefs that can be tested empirically. For example, one associated belief is that as many healthcare issues have important ethical as well as technical dimensions, involving the public may help ensure health policy decisions better reflect the values of the community. This belief could be tested by assessing how far the mechanisms for involving the public help to reach a generally accepted view on an ethical dilemma.

A second argument for increasing public involvement is that it will make services more responsive to the individuals and communities who use them and that more responsive services will lead to improved health. Underpinning these assumptions is the belief that professional definitions of benefit in health care can be at best only partial; only the users or local communities themselves know what they need, and it is ultimately their assessment of benefit that matters.

Who should be consulted?

Returning to the article by Lomas that you read earlier in the chapter, another main issue raised by the author was which members of the public should be consulted. You have seen one approach (Bowling, 1996) – surveys of large, randomly selected samples of the population. For many countries, the expense of such an approach has led to the exploration of other methods. One example was to see if the views of community leaders could substitute for more widespread consultation. Obinna Onwujekwe and colleagues (1999) compared the views of community leaders in three areas of Nigeria with the views of local people regarding the financing and distribution of drugs to treat onchocerciasis (river blindness). They found that while there was no significant difference in relation to the method of collecting payments, managing and making payments, who should set the level of payments, and the drug distribution mechanisms, there were differences concerning how the scheme should be supervised.

The extract below outlines their conclusion:

Can community leaders' preferences be used to proxy those of the community as a whole?

It appears that one can never completely substitute preferences elicited from households with those of community leaders, as there are likely to be some points of disagreement between the two classes of people. However, bearing time and resource constraints in mind, one approach would be to collect information from community leaders during surveys and then discuss the results in general assemblies of communities, so that areas of conflict could be resolved before programme implementation.

The findings also show the importance of conducting a comparative analysis in different areas of the preferences of both community leaders and heads of households before mounting community-based health care interventions. Such an approach should help to discover whether and, if so where, there are disparities between the views of community leaders and heads of households and whether these vary between areas, in order to resolve any differences during the planning stage of any initiative. It is now well established from other research that people's own words and experiences bring into sharp focus the problems that influence their satisfaction with health care, and that addressing these problems by allowing community voices to be heard and affirming the importance of their experience for health care planning is essential in ensuring that widely available and efficacious primary health care interventions become effective in practice.

Summary

Users of health services play multiple roles and these roles have been changing over time, with increasing levels of participation in the decision-making processes relating to the services provided and personal care. However, countries differ in the levels of user engagement and even in high-income contexts it is unclear to what extent there is real citizen power.

You have seen that good staff–patient communication is critical for patient satisfaction and outcome of care. Various factors have been found to influence the style of interaction with patients. Research suggests that key aspects of a successful encounter include eliciting the full range of patients' concerns, being empathic, and delivering adequate information. Training of health professionals in interpersonal skills helps to improve staff–patient interaction. The distribution of relative power in the staff–patient relationship is shaped by various factors, including cultural norms and the bureaucratic organization of health services.

Various initiatives have been designed to transfer power to users of health services. They have involved better information, improved handling of complaints, advocacy schemes, the representation of consumers at various levels of health services, and mechanisms protecting patients' rights. Finally, this chapter has examined the relevance of consumerism for health care and the ways in which users as citizens and community might be more involved in decisions about services and policy.

References

Arnstein, S.R. (1969) A ladder of citizen participation, *American Institute of Planners Journal*, 35 (4): 216–24.
Aronson, J.K. (2007) Compliance, concordance, adherence, *British Journal of Clinical Pharmacology*, 63 (4): 383–4.

Bernhart, M., Wiadyana, I.G.P., Wihardjo, H. and Pohan, I. (1999) Patient satisfaction in developing countries, *Social Science and Medicine*, 48 (8): 989–96.

Berwick, D.M. (2009) What 'patient-centred' should mean: confessions of an extremist, *Health Affairs (Millwood)*, 28 (4): 555–65.

Bhat, R. (1996) Regulating the private health care sector: the case of the Indian Consumer Protection Act, *Health Policy and Planning*, 11 (3): 265–79.

Bowling, A. (1996) Health care rationing: the public's debate, *British Medical Journal*, 312 (7032): 670–4.

Chowdhury, A.M., Chowdhury, S., Islam, M.N., Islam, A. and Vaughan, J.P. (1997) Control of tuberculosis by community health workers in Bangladesh, *Lancet*, 350 (9072): 169–72.

Cooper, L., Coote, A., Davies, A. and Jackson, C. (1995) *Voices Off: Tackling the democratic deficit in health*. London: Institute of Public Policy Research.

Coulter, A. (2002) *The Autonomous Patient*. London: TSO.

Crawford, M.J., Rutter, D., Manley, C., Weaver, T., Bhui, K., Fulop, N. et al. (2002) Systematic review of involving patients in the planning and development of health care, *British Medical Journal*, 325 (7375): 1263–8.

Donaldson, L. (2003) Expert patients usher in a new era of opportunity for the NHS, *British Medical Journal*, 326 (7402): 1279–80.

Egbert, L.D., Battit, G.E., Welch, C.E. and Bartlett, M.K. (1964) Reduction of post-operative pain by encouragement and instruction of patients: a study of doctor–patient rapport, *New England Journal of Medicine*, 270: 825–7.

Florin, D. and Dixon, J. (2004) Public involvement in health care, *British Medical Journal*, 328 (7432): 159–61.

Levinson, W., Roter, D.L., Mullooly, J.P., Dull, V.T. and Frankel, R.M. (1997) Physician–patient communication: the relationship with malpractice claims among primary care physicians and surgeons, *Journal of the American Medical Association*, 277 (7): 553–9.

Lomas, J. (1997). Reluctant rationers: public input to health care priorities, *Journal of Health Services Research and Policy*, 2 (2): 103–11.

Lorig, K.R., Sobel, D.S., Stewart, A.L., Brown, B.W., Jr., Bandura, A., Ritter, P. et al. (1999) Evidence suggesting that a chronic disease self-management program can improve health status while reducing hospitalization: a randomised trial, *Medical Care*, 37 (1): 5–14.

Lupton, D. (1997) Consumerism, reflexivity and the medical encounter, *Social Science and Medicine*, 45 (3): 373–81.

Mol, A. (2008) *The Logic of Care: Health and the problem of patient choice*. London: Routledge.

Nettleton, S. and Harding, S. (1994) Protesting patients: a study of complaints submitted to a Family Health Services Authority, *Sociology of Health and Illness*, 16 (1): 38–63.

Onwujekwe, O., Shu, E. and Okonkwo, P. (1999) Can community leaders' preferences be used to proxy those of the community as a whole?, *Journal of Health Services Research and Policy*, 4 (3): 133–8.

Parsons, T. (1951) *The Social System*. Glencoe, IL: Free Press.

Parsons, T. and Mayhew, L.H. (eds) (1982) *On Institutions and Social Evolution: Selected writings*. Chicago, IL: University of Chicago Press.

Rusmiyati, R. (1997) *Focus Group Discussions for Developing a Patient Satisfaction Questionnaire*. Jakarta: Directorate of Health Center Development, Ministry of Health.

Saltman, R.B. (1994) Patient choice and patient empowerment in northern European health systems: a conceptual framework, *International Journal of Health Services*, 24 (2): 210–29.

Saltman, R.B. and Figueras, J. (eds) (1997) *European Health Care Reform: Analysis of current strategies*. Copenhagen: WHO Regional Office for Europe.

Sbaro, J.A. and Sbaro, J.B. (1994) Compliance and supervision of chemotherapy of tuberculosis, *Seminars in Respiratory Infections*, 9 (2): 120–7.

Sinyor, J.K. (1997) *Pregnant Women's Satisfaction with Antenatal Care.* Jakarta: Directorate of Health Center Development, Ministry of Health.

Weber, M. (1922/1958) Bureaucracy, in H.H. Gerth (ed. and trans.) *From Max Weber: Essays in sociology.* Oxford: Oxford University Press.

Williams, S.J. and Calnan, M. (1991) Key determinants of consumer satisfaction with general practice, *Family Practice,* 8 (3): 237–42.

World Health Organization (WHO) (2015) *Tuberculosis,* Fact sheet #104. Revised March 2015. Geneva: WHO.

9 Paying providers

Overview

This chapter discusses the issue of asymmetric information in health care markets and how it modifies the agency relationship. It then identifies and explains the main provider payment methods typically used to pay individual practitioners and organizations, and the incentives created by these mechanisms.

Learning objectives

After working through this chapter, you will be able to:

- describe the agency relationship in health care markets
- describe the main provider payment methods for individual practitioners and medical institutions
- explain the various incentives created by these payment mechanisms and their potential impact on the quantity, quality, and costs of health care

Key terms

Agency theory (or principal-agent theory): Describes the problems that arise under conditions of asymmetric information between two parties, the principal and the agent.

Capitation payment: A predetermined amount of money per member of a defined population served by the third party payer, given to a provider to deliver specific services.

DRG (Diagnosis Related Group)/HRG (Healthcare Resource Group): A case-mix classification scheme that provides a means of relating the number and type of acute in-patients treated in a hospital to the resources required by the hospital.

Fee-for-service: Payment mechanism whereby providers receive a specific amount of money for each service provided.

Agency relationship

Agency relationship is a theory used by economists as well as other social scientists as a way to describe the relationship between two parties: the principal and the agent. The principal is a person who delegates responsibilities to agents to act on their behalf. The primary issue in the relationship between the principal and agent is an information asymmetry problem: agents have greater access to strategic information or technical skills than principals and principals cannot observe agents' efforts or performance. Payment mechanisms can create incentives that will align the interests of the principal and those of the agent (Lagarde, 2011).

✎ Activity 9.1

Think about the relationship between the patient, the doctor, and the payer. There are two agency relationships here. The first is between the patient and the doctor; the second is between the payer and the doctor. Who are the principal and the agent in these relationships? What is the principal's problem that needs to be delegated? Why does the information asymmetry arise? In what ways would the information asymmetry impact the amount or the quality of health care provided?

Feedback

In the patient–doctor relationship, the principal is the patient and the doctor is the agent. When sick, people consult doctors to act on their behalf and prescribe the best course of treatment. The information asymmetry arises as patients lack medical knowledge to specify what treatments need to be carried out or judge whether doctors do the right thing or not. Doctors, on the other hand, possess the knowledge and the legal authority to treat health problems and prescribe medication. Normally, agents are expected to act to maximize their own utility, but due to the nature of health care markets doctors might have other potentially diverging objectives. For example, while doctors would care about improving patients' benefits and welfare, they may wish to do that while minimizing their efforts and maximizing their income. In Chapter 6, you learnt that providers are able to induce demand if their income is related to it, such as by advising more tests even though they are unnecessary. There might also be a lack of effort or lower quality of care, as all things being equal, providers will minimize their efforts for a given level of remuneration. A further complication of doctor–patient agency relationship is that even if the doctor has been a good 'agent', providing appropriate and high quality care, there is significant uncertainty associated with medical care and the doctor's efforts might not be sufficient to restore a patient to good health. Therefore, it is very difficult to determine whether the doctor met the principal's expectations and represented the principal's interests.

The second relationship is between the payer and the provider. Third-party payers (such as insurance companies, health care authorities, and hospitals) hire doctors to provide care to their beneficiaries (patients). The principal's main concern here is whether the resources are used in an efficient way while providing good quality care. The agents (doctors), in addition to the divergent objectives discussed above, also need to think about complying with what their managers are telling them to do. The information asymmetry arises as the third-party payers cannot observe doctors' efforts and whether doctors' decisions are made in an efficient and appropriate manner.

Thomas Rice notes that doctors are in fact 'not double but quadruple' agents: for the patient, for themselves, for the insurer that pays for the service, and for society as a whole. Each of these has its own set of objectives that need to be fulfilled, and it is very unlikely that a doctor would be able to maximize all four sets of utility functions with one set of actions (Rice, 2006).

A typology for payment mechanisms

A simple typology of reimbursing health care practitioners and institutions, proposed by Tim Ensor and Jack Langenbrunner, relates to whether payment is time-based, service-based or population-based (Ensor and Langenbrunner, 2002). With time-based payment, providers are paid according to the length of time spent providing the service, irrespective of the number of patients served. Service-based payment depends on the number of services provided or patients treated and can be categorized on the basis of unit of service (ranging from basic units of service such as visits, diagnostic tests or hospital days, to bundles of services or patient episodes). Population-based remuneration is payment according to the size of the population served by the facility, irrespective of the numbers of patients actually attending. Most types of payment can be categorized under one of these groups (Table 9.1).

Historically, for many countries in Europe and North America, provider remuneration was mainly time- and population-based. For example, staff were paid a salary that was fixed irrespective of the level of work or size of the population catchment area. The payments were based on input characteristics such as past qualifications and years of experience for individual providers, and beds and staff for facilities. These approaches, however, did not allow for flexibility to respond to local needs, changes in technology or treatment patterns. Many countries therefore have moved away or are

Table 9.1 Types of payment mechanisms

	Individual practitioner	Medical institution
Time-based	Salary	Fixed budget (based usually on historic allocations)
Services-based	Fee-for-service Fee for patient episode (e.g. admission) Target payments	Fee-for-service Fee per hospital day (per diem) Fee for patient episode Budget based on case-mix/utilization
Population-based	Per capita payment, territorial payment	Block contract

Source: Ensor and Langenbrunner (2002).

transitioning from input-based budgets and salaries for providers towards payments that are linked to services, outputs, and ultimately outcomes (Langenbrunner et al., 2005). While a mix of payment methods is often the most effective way of optimizing the positive and negative incentives on individual or hospital behaviours, capacity constraints in low- and middle-income countries may preclude complex combinations of payment mechanisms (McIntyre, 2007), and time- and population-based approaches remain the predominant payment method in many countries. You will now explore how these payment mechanisms create provider incentives that can impact the quantity, quality, and costs of care provided.

Paying individual practitioners

The main forms of payment mechanisms for individual practitioners are salary, fee-for-service, and capitation payment.

Salary

Under salary arrangements, the provider is paid a fixed amount over a particular period of time. The payments are determined prospectively and paid retrospectively. The amount could be linked to a number of hours of work, but it is not linked to number of services provided or patients. Administrative costs of maintaining a salary-based provider payment system are low, and the expenditures are predictable. Salary payments to individual providers are used in many countries, especially in the public sector.

The main advantage of salary payments is that there is no incentive to deliver unnecessary services or to induce demand. However, there might be an incentive for 'under-provision', to the extent that providers may attempt to work less (and provide fewer services) than expected in their contract. Salaried payment systems have been found to be associated with lower levels of health services (measured by tests, procedures, and referrals) when compared with systems with other payment mechanisms (fee-for-service and capitation) (Gosden et al., 1999).

The disadvantage of salary payments is that there is little incentive for efficient behaviour and for the individual providers to deliver high quality care or be responsive to patients' demands and expectations. There is some scope to reward effort or good quality of care using payment increments or promotions, and typically there is a reliance on peer-review of practices and enforcement of rules and procedures thought to enhance quality. This could indeed improve quality or if the rule enforcement limits professional judgement in treatment decisions, it might result in a lower quality of care (Christianson et al., 2007).

Fee-for-service

Fee-for-service is paying providers for volume of services provided. There are different variants of fee-for-service, the extreme version of which itemizes each service. The fee schedule is known and negotiated between the payer and the provider. Fee-for-service is common in many high-income countries, and in particular in the private sector, although use of fee-for-service in the public sector can also be seen in France and Germany (for semi-private GP and specialist services).

The positive incentives created by fee-for-service include increased motivation and efforts of providers; it can also be used in some cases to increase the volume of under-provided services, in particular for those services that are provided regularly (e.g. immunization). The main disadvantage is that fee-for-service creates incentives for the provider to increase the volume or induce demand of services where the fee is higher than the cost of providing the service (including physician time), generating additional revenue for the provider. This also implies that fee-for-service will on average result in higher health care spending for the payers and society as a whole, and may require a substantial amount of monitoring by the payer. The administrative costs of fee-for-service-based payment mechanisms are also high.

While the expected impact of fee-for-service on quantity of services is quite clear, its anticipated effect on quality is not. It can be argued that fee-for-service would not have a detrimental impact on quality of care or patient outcomes because the providers do not have an incentive to withhold services and that more health care would benefit patients in most cases. However, physician income increases regardless of whether the provided services are needed or not, and a growing literature suggests that there is a risk to patient health associated with 'over-treatment', just as there is with 'under-treatment' (Christianson et al., 2007).

Capitation payment

Capitation payment is the most complex payment mechanisms to set up, where the provider agrees to deliver a specified list of health services to a predetermined group of individuals (such as patients in their catchment area or list) for a fixed amount per person per time period. The provider therefore bears the financial risk in situations for which the actual cost of these services exceeds the fixed payment. Capitation rate is set and paid prospectively and can be adjusted by the socio-demographic/health status of the population served (e.g. the rates for young children and the elderly who are more likely to use health services are higher than that of young adults). The capitation payment mechanism is used for GPs in several countries, including the UK, Italy, and Spain.

With capitation payments, as with salaries, there is no problem of supplier-induced demand. However, in contrast to salaries, capitation payments encourage provider competition to attract patients. If the provider has any control over the population to be served, there is also an incentive to select or enrol healthier patients ('cream-skimming'), particularly if capitation rates are not properly adjusted for the case-mix.

With capitation payments, there might be an economic incentive to provide as little care as possible per patient, while aiming to maximize the number of patients cared for. While under-provision of services could in the short term increase income for providers, this strategy is likely to be unsustainable because patients may choose other providers if they feel that the provider is not responsive to their needs and expectations. If the provider eliminates some necessary as well as some 'unnecessary' services in an effort to reduce service use, this would also result in a lower quality of care and poorer outcomes for patients. These 'aggressive' constraints on service use are more likely if there is no sharing of risk or surplus, if the capitated contract is short term, and its renewal only depends on costs (Christianson et al., 2007). However, capitation payments also provide incentives that are potentially quality-enhancing: if patients are free to choose their providers, competition might drive up the quality of the services to attract more patients and there is also an increased emphasis on preventative services to ensure the population cared for remains as healthy as possible.

Paying institutions

The main forms of payment mechanisms for institutions are line-item budgets, fee-for-service, per diem, case-based payment, and global budget allocations.

Line-item budgets

Line-item budgets are prospective payments to cover operating costs of providing services, based on projected input use. These include specification of the number and type of staff employed in the hospital and non-salary expenditures, which are determined by past patterns of input or government regulations on the level and composition of inputs used (Schneider, 2008).

Line-item budgeting is a good method to control costs, providing predictable budgets and expenses while ensuring a minimum standard in each facility. It is administratively simple and a low-cost mechanism to set up, with limited need for information systems. However, it does not create incentives for efficient management of resources or provision of high quality health services that are responsive to patient needs. It is inefficient because there is often little or no flexibility in reallocating the line-items to adapt to local circumstances. Institutions also have a tendency to create high levels of fixed resources, increase the numbers of staff and beds, and sustain excess capacity as the budget is tied to these inputs. Health care is more likely to be rationed or under-provided with line-item budgets, with institutions having incentives to refer high-risk patients to other providers.

Most public hospitals in Western and Central Europe were paid fixed line-budgets prior to the hospital payment reform in the mid-1980s. The countries of Eastern Europe and Central Asia (notably, former Soviet Union countries) also used this type of hospital payment mechanism, as it allowed for a strong central control when management skills in local regions were inadequate. Typically, the number and type of staff were determined by the number of beds in an in-patient setting, and by the size of the population for a polyclinic. Total staffing budget was obtained by multiplying the number of staff by the national pay scale, which was based on specialty and experience, with some further adjustment (e.g. for geographical region). Funding for other items was based on the facility and population-specific norms; for example, hospital food expenditures were based on the number of bed-days in the previous year (Ensor and Langenbrunner, 2002). Many countries have since developed or are developing payment systems that pay for a defined unit of hospital output.

Fee-for-service

With fee-for-service payments, the institutions are reimbursed based on the number or procedures or services they provide. As discussed earlier, while fee-for-service payments guarantee access to care (as well as provision of the 'best care available', if the price of the item exceeds the costs), they also create incentives to perform more procedures, which is likely to increase health expenditures and possibly have an adverse effect on quality of care. Jegers and colleagues note that composing the list of reimbursable medical activities and in particular determining the relative value of each item involve a 'complex and delicate process', with 'technical procedures often being overvalued relative to intellectual acts'. There might be further misallocation of resources if the relative value of items does not follow the evolution in the actual costs and benefits of technological developments and remains unchanged for long periods (Jegers et al., 2002).

An example of a country that used fee-for-service for hospital payments is the Czech Republic in the early 1990s. In 1993, there were 27 non-profit

insurance companies, paying providers on a purely fee-for-service schedule of 5000 services. The volume of services and expenditures grew rapidly, with the expenditures increasing by 46 per cent until 1995, when the
expenditures were capped. Companies began to go bankrupt from 1995,
and only nine remained by 1998, leaving significant unpaid debts. The
remaining insurers shifted to new payment systems (Langenbrunner and
Wiley, 2002).

Payment per patient-day

With the 'per-diem' reimbursement system, the facility receives a set amount
of payment per bed-day. With per-diem payments, there is an incentive to
increase admissions and length of hospitalizations beyond that necessary
(if the marginal cost of providing hospital services is less than the per-diem
rate) and rationing of resource use to stay within the payment and increase
surplus per day. In these systems, specialists play a decisive role in hospital reimbursement because they determine the length of stay of patients
by their admission and discharge policy. The providers are also likely to aim
to attract healthier patients or avoid costly patients.

This payment mechanism was introduced in some Eastern European countries in the transition years of the early 1990s, as it did not require much
data and capacity to design or implement but could promote productivity and
increase revenues for hospitals. Initially, the payment rates were determined
by recurrent costs (not including capital costs or depreciation) and basic
case-mix adjustment (e.g. department of facility). Overall expenditure caps,
other case-mix or facility adjusters, and mixed payment methods (such as
points systems for providers or fee-for-service for some procedures) were
used to supplement the basic per-diem payments in some countries (e.g.
Croatia, Slovakia, Slovenia, Estonia) (Langenbrunner et al., 2005).

Payment per case

With case-based payments, the facility receives a set amount per
discharge or per case. With simple case-based models, the payment is
based on a fixed payment by discharge regardless of the type of case
and the actual cost of care. As in per-diem payments, from a payer perspective these payments improve the efficient use of resources because
the providers will have incentives to stay within costs. This may lead to
increased admissions when the case payment is higher than the actual
cost per case; for example, hospitals may admit a patient who could be
treated more efficiently in an out-patient or day-surgery setting. It can
also lead to rationing of resource use and patient selection to increase
surplus per case.

To improve hospital efficiency, and using techniques from industrial
management, Fetter and colleagues identified ways in which inputs could

be linked to hospital outputs (Fetter, 1991). With case-based payments adjusted for case-mix, the facility receives a set amount per hospitalization, but more complex cases attract higher funding and in some settings the payments are further adjusted for facility characteristics and local costs. This reimbursement method is very popular for hospitals, and most high-income countries have introduced such systems. For example, in the USA, the complexity of the case is identified through 467 classes of patients or diagnosis-related groups (DRGs), grouped according to clinically similar treatments and expected resource use during their hospital stay. In the UK, a similar system using healthcare resource groups (HRGs) is used. Similar case-based payment systems have been introduced in some middle-income countries, including Korea, Taiwan, Thailand, and Hungary (Langenbrunner et al., 2005).

In theory, DRG-based payment systems create incentives to reduce costs per treated patient, to increase revenues per patient, and to increase the number of patients (Cots et al., 2011). Hospital strategies to reduce costs per treated patient include reducing length of stay (e.g. by optimizing internal care pathways, transferring to other providers, and inappropriate early discharge), reducing the intensity of provided services (e.g. by avoiding delivering unnecessary services, substituting high-cost services with low-cost alternatives or withholding necessary services – 'skimping/under-treatment'), and patient selection (e.g. by specializing in treating patients for which the hospital has a competitive advantage or selecting low-cost patients). Hospitals can aim to increase revenue per patient by changing coding practices (e.g. by improving coding of diagnoses and procedures or by fraudulent reclassification of patients through adding non-existent secondary diagnoses) or changing practice patterns (e.g. by providing services that lead to reclassification of patients into higher-paying DRGs). Increasing the number of patients can be possible by changing admission rules (e.g. by reducing the waiting list, splitting care episodes into multiple admissions, admitting patients for unnecessary services) or improving the reputation of the hospital through improving the quality of services or focusing efforts exclusively on measurable areas. Depending on the payment system and relative strength of these incentives, these strategies might improve or reduce the quality and efficiency of health services.

Activity 9.2

Richard Busse and colleagues (2013) reviewed the experience of DRG-based payments in 12 European countries. As you read the excerpt from their article below, note the incentives that are created by case-based systems and their intended and unintended consequences. How can these unintended consequences be avoided or reduced?

Diagnosis related groups in Europe: moving towards transparency, efficiency, and quality in hospitals?

... In Europe most countries developed their own DRG systems in the 1990s (though Portugal started in the early 1980s). Some developed their systems from scratch (Austria, England, the Netherlands); others imported a DRG system from abroad and used it as the starting point for developing their own. Only Ireland, Portugal, and Spain continue to use imported systems from the US or Australia. The Nordic countries have created a common system.

... Because most countries in Europe moved to DRG-based payment from global budgets, their experience differs from that in the US, where DRG-based payments succeeded fee for service. In the US the introduction of DRG-based payments initially led to a reduction in hospital activity; the effect (as intended) in Europe was an increase in activity, particularly in day care. For example, in England between 2003 and 2007, day care activity increased by about 15% while total NHS inpatient activity increased by 10%. While in the US DRG-based payment helped contain costs, the increase in activity in Europe mostly led to higher hospital costs. For example, in Austria between 1997 and 2007, total hospital costs increased by 3.8% annually, while costs per case increased by 1.7%. Whether increased activity and reduced costs per case led to improved efficiency in European hospitals and whether this was the direct effect of DRG-based payment are difficult to say.

DRG-based hospital payment may have unintended consequences if the effects are too strong. For example, DRG-based payments are intended to reduce length of stay and cost of treatment, but an excessive reduction in length of stay may reduce the quality of care. Research in Europe found little change in death rates and readmissions when DRG-based hospital payments were introduced. However, in France 30-day readmission rates after discharge seem to have increased since the introduction of DRG-based payment and a study from Sweden showed that patient-perceived quality of care decreased.

Other potential unintended consequences of DRG-based hospital payment include cherry picking, dumping, upcoding, overtreatment, and frequent readmissions. Cherry picking occurs if certain patients within one group are systematically more costly than others, leading to incentives for hospitals to select the less costly, more profitable cases and to transfer or avoid the unprofitable ones ('dumping'). Upcoding refers to hospitals increasing their revenue by coding additional diagnoses to move patients into a higher-paying group. Furthermore, hospitals may even change their practice patterns, providing procedures that place patients in higher-paying groups (such as treating patients with acute myocardial infarction with drug eluting stents instead of bare metal stents); or they could admit or readmit patients to hospital for unnecessary services or for *conditions that could be treated in outpatients (currently few countries use DRG-based payments for outpatient activity and inpatient treatment may be more profitable).*

Our research in Europe suggests that these unintended consequences are relatively rare – or at least that they have been detected rarely despite (or because of) regular audits by monitoring and review bodies. Evidence of cherry picking is available only for England and France, where private providers have been found to treat less complex patients than public hospitals. Intentional upcoding and overtreatment are substantial problems in France and Germany but seem to be uncommon elsewhere.

Several countries have introduced policies to try to prevent frequent readmissions and overtreatment. For example, in Germany and England, hospitals are – under certain conditions – not paid for readmissions within 30 days from the initial admission or discharge. Furthermore, to avoid an excessive increase in the number of admissions, hospitals in England in 2013 receive only 30% of the full tariff for emergency admissions that exceed the number of admissions in the financial year 2008–09. Similarly, in Germany, total hospital activity is limited by negotiated target budgets and hospitals can keep only 35% of the revenue earned for activity provided in excess of the budget.

From Busse, R. et al. (2013) Diagnosis related groups in Europe: moving towards transparency, efficiency, and quality in hospitals?, *British Medical Journal*, 346:f3197, with permission from BMJ Publishing Group Ltd.

Feedback

European experiences with DRGs were characterized by higher levels of activity (particularly in day care) and, in most cases, increased overall costs. The authors also noted incentives in some countries to 'game the system' and increase revenues by patient selection, overtreatment or frequent readmissions, and changing coding practices.

Cots and colleagues note three broad strategies that have been used to avoid the unintended consequences in Europe (Cots et al., 2011). The first one is to improve the fairness of payment by assuring adequate payment for outliers and high-cost services. If DRG systems use high quality data on costs and are good at creating groups of patients that have similar costs while adequately controlling for the differences between patients and treatments, incentives for patient selection and undertreatment would be reduced. If DRGs are very narrowly defined, however, providers are likely to use other strategies such as changing their coding practice. Although DRG systems are continuously refined to improve these consequences, additional measures are required for high-cost 'outlier' cases, which give hospitals strong incentives to avoid these high-cost cases or to discharge them inappropriately early. Most of the countries in Europe have developed mechanisms to identify outlier cases and to pay hospitals separately for the extra costs of treating such patients. The second broad strategy is to monitor and control these unintended consequences, such as through regular audits by monitoring and review bodies, as noted in the text. Some countries have also used financial mechanisms to control cost and levels of activity, for example, by determining global budgets or volume thresholds to ensure that hospitals do not increase their activity beyond predetermined limits. The third broad strategy is to decrease the relative power of DRG incentives by reducing the share of DRG-based payment in total hospital revenues.

Busse and colleagues highlight that countries are moving towards DRG-based payment systems that are extended to day care and outpatient settings, and those that also provide incentives for improving quality. These developments are likely to further improve the unintended consequences of DRG-based payment systems (Busse et al., 2013).

Global budgets

With global budgets, the facility receives a prospective lump-sum payment to cover the expected expenditures over a given period to provide a set of services that have been broadly agreed upon. They are often implemented in response to volume problems under per diem and per case payment systems and have been used in many European countries and Canada.

A global budget may be based on either inputs or outputs, or a combination of the two (Langenbrunner et al., 2005) and in its simplest form, calculated using historical budgets or utilization, with more complex systems also adjusting for the case-mix of the population covered (e.g. by age/sex, morbidity or social equity factors). Therefore, this payment mechanism depends on the availability of comprehensive cost and activity data. Similar to other types of budgets, it constrains the growth of price and quantity of services. However, unlike line-item budgets, it also gives flexibility to use and allocate the budget across services as appropriate and allows for local management autonomy. The surplus could be kept by the facility but expenditures over budgetary allocation must be sourced from elsewhere. The pressure to keep the costs within the budgetary boundaries encourages the facilities to use resources effectively but might also provide incentives to lower the quality of care or ration services (Langenbrunner and Wiley, 2002).

Paying for performance

New provider payment methods are being developed or implemented better to align payment incentives with objectives relevant to promoting health service quality, care coordination, health improvement, and efficiency by rewarding achievement of performance measures (Cashin et al., 2014). There is no widely accepted definition of pay for performance (P4P), and the term is often used interchangeably with other terms such as 'performance-based funding', 'paying for results', and 'results-based financing'. Definitions reflecting perspectives from early schemes in the USA focus on quality improvement, while more recent definitions concerning low- and middle-income country perspectives are broader to include both incentives on the supply side to providers and also demand-side incentives (such as conditional cash transfers). Although there are differences in terminology, all P4P programme designs include four common elements: performance domains and measures (e.g. clinical quality, coverage, efficiency, and their indicators), the basis for reward or penalty (e.g. targets, changes in measure over time or relative ranking), the reward or penalty (e.g. bonus payments or non-financial incentives), and the data reporting and verification processes. Depending on the objectives of the programme, there are a variety of choices that could be made for each element (Cashin, 2014).

Cashin and colleagues (2014) reviewed the experiences from P4P schemes in OECD countries. In 2012, P4P programmes on payments to providers were reported in 15 OECD countries, focusing on primary care physicians (15), specialists (8), and hospitals (8). For individual physicians, most of these schemes involved bonus payments for reaching performance targets such as preventive care, efficiency of care, patient satisfaction, and management of chronic diseases. For hospitals, some programmes include bonuses or penalties, mostly for processes of care, but some also for clinical outcomes and patient satisfaction (Cashin, 2014). A review of P4P schemes in low- and middle-income countries identified three broad approaches to incentivizing quality, which are used in combination in most countries (Ergo et al., 2012). The first approach involves rewards for attaining accreditation standards. For example, in Brazil, hospitals associated with one large private, non-profit health insurer are paid increased per-diem rates for initiating and achieving successive levels of quality accreditation. A second approach involves rewards for achieving performance on quality components incorporated in correct treatment protocols. For example, Benin's nationwide scheme rewards providers for timely and justified referral for complicated deliveries and for other performance indicators relevant to child growth monitoring and postnatal care. While these indicators are relatively easy to collect and understand, they are narrow in focus and it is often difficult to monitor overall quality of care provided at the facility. In the third approach, some countries are exploring the use of quality checklists or scorecards and the calculation of a quality index or score, which is then used to adjust the performance payment that a health facility should receive based on the quantity of services delivered. Rwanda is one of the first countries to incorporate such a checklist in its nationwide scheme. Rwanda's P4P scheme and two other examples from the UK and the USA are discussed in detail in Box 9.1.

Box 9.1 Examples of P4P schemes

USA: Premier Ltd Hospital Quality Incentive Demonstration (PHQID)

In the United States, the development of large-scale P4P pilot or demonstration projects through Medicare & Medicaid Services was initiated after the publication of the Institute of Medicine's *Crossing the Quality Chasm* report (Institute of Medicine, 2001), which suggested that effective health care reform could come from influencing provider payment mechanisms (Ergo et al., 2012). PHQID was a large pilot providing bonus payments to hospitals (Medicare patients) based on a composite measure of in-patient quality for specific conditions. Hospitals performing in the top (second) decile on a composite measure of quality receive a 2 per cent (1 per cent) bonus payment in addition to usual Medicare reimbursement rates. The programme also implemented penalties for a hospital's failure to achieve benchmarks. Evidence on PHQID indicates a positive but small impact on quality of care but not on health outcomes or on costs (Ryan, 2009).

UK: Quality and Outcomes Framework

The Quality and Outcomes Framework (QOF) was introduced in the UK in 2004 as part of the new general practitioner contract that remunerates performance against a multitude of quality-of-care indicators. The programme primarily aimed to improve the management of common chronic conditions, such as diabetes and stroke, in primary care. It is one of the world's largest pay-for-performance schemes of its kind, at a cost of approximately £1 billion a year. The payments are based on complex calculations: providers are awarded points on a sliding scale on the basis of the proportion of eligible patients for whom the target is achieved. No points are awarded over a maximum threshold. Targets are based on four different domains: clinical, organizational, patient experience and additional services. There is some evidence that QOF has incentivized general practices to have a more organized approach to chronic disease management, and provide an incentive to engage in secondary prevention. However, there were overall no incentives for primary prevention and undertaking public health activities (Dixon et al., 2011). There were improvements in quality of care for two of three chronic conditions in the short term. However, once targets were reached, the improvement in the quality of care for patients with these conditions slowed (Campbell et al., 2009). There was limited impact on non-incentivized activities, with adverse effects reported for some specific sub-populations, such as older patients and patients in deprived areas (Langdown and Peckham, 2014).

Rwanda: Performance-Based Financing National Programme (Basinga et al., 2011)

The Rwandan national scheme was set up in 2005 to provide bonus payments to primary health providers based on the quantity and quality of priority health services. The P4P payments are linked to 14 key maternal and child health care output indicators, including visit and outreach indicators (such as number of prenatal visits) and content of care indicators (such as tetanus vaccination during prenatal care). This payment is multiplied by a quality of care index to calculate the amount of money the facility will receive through the P4P scheme. The index is based on structural and process-related measures of quality derived from Rwandan clinical practice guidelines. Structural measures assess the extent to which the facility has the equipment, drugs, medical supplies, and personnel necessary to deliver a specific medical service, whereas process measures rate the clinical content of care actually provided for services. The evidence from an impact evaluation of the programme suggested increased rates of institutional delivery care and child health visits, but no impact of P4P payments on prenatal care visits or immunization rates. The authors concluded that the scheme in Rwanda had the greatest effect on services that had the highest payment rates and needed the least effort from the service provider.

Summary

In this chapter, you have explored a wide range of payment methods for individual providers and hospitals. Each payment mechanism creates a set of incentives that influence provider behaviour, but often there is a trade-off between the provision of good quality care and efficient use of resources. Most health systems will therefore use a blend of these mechanisms to pay providers and an increasing number of new provider payment mechanism are being developed or implemented globally to explicitly reward providers for delivering better quality care.

References

Basinga, P., Gertler, P.J., Binagwaho, A., Soucat, A.L., Sturdy, J. and Vermeersch, C.M. (2011) Effect on maternal and child health services in Rwanda of payment to primary health-care providers for performance: an impact evaluation, *Lancet*, 377 (775): 1421–8.

Busse, R., Geissler, A., Aaviksoo, A., Cots, F., Häkkinen, U., Kobel, C. et al. (2013) Diagnosis related groups in Europe: moving towards transparency, efficiency, and quality in hospitals?, *British Medical Journal*, 346: f3197.

Campbell, S.M., Reeves, D., Kontopantelis, E., Sibbsald, B. and Roland, M. (2009) Effects of pay for performance on the quality of primary care in England, *New England Journal of Medicine*, 361: 368–78.

Cashin, C. (2014) P4P Programme design, in C. Cashin, Y.L. Chi, P.C. Smith, M. Borowitz and S. Thomson (eds) *Paying for Performance in Health Care: Implications for health system performance and accountability*. Maidenhead: Open University Press.

Cashin, C., Chi, Y.L., Smith, P.C., Borowitz, M. and Thomson, S. (2014) Health provider P4P and strategic health purchasing, in C. Cashin, Y.L. Chi, P.C. Smith, M. Borowitz and S. Thomson (eds) *Paying for Performance in Health Care: Implications for health system performance and accountability*. Maidenhead: Open University Press.

Christianson, J.B., Leatherman, S. and Sutherland, K. (2007) *Financial Incentives, Healthcare Providers and Quality Improvements: A review of the evidence*. London: The Health Foundation.

Cots, F., Chiarello, P., Salvador, X. and Quentin, W. (2011) DRG-based hospital payment: intended and unintended consequences, in R. Busse, A. Geissler, W. Quentin and M. Wiley (eds) *Diagnosis-Related Groups in Europe: Moving towards transparency, efficiency and quality in hospitals*. Maidenhead: Open University Press.

Dixon, A., Khachatryan, A., Wallace, A., Peckham, S., Boyce, T. and Gillam, S. (2011) *Impact of Quality and Outcomes Framework on Health Inequalities*. London: The King's Fund.

Ensor, T. and Langenbrunner, J. (2002) Allocating resources and paying providers, in M. McKee, J. Healy and J. Falkingham (eds) *Health Care in Central Asia*. Buckingham: Open University Press.

Ergo, A., Paina, L., Morgan, L. and Eichler, R. (2012) *Creating Stronger Incentives for High-Quality Health Care in Low- and Middle-Income Countries*. Washington, DC: USAID Maternal and Child Health Integrated Program.

Fetter, R.B. (ed.) (1991) *DRGs: Their design and development*. Ann Arbor, MI: Health Administration Press.

Gosden, T., Pedersen, L. and Torgerson, D. (1999) How should we pay doctors? A systematic review of salary payments and their effect on doctor behavior, *QJM: An International Journal of Medicine*, 92 (1): 47–55.

Institute of Medicine (2001) *Crossing the Quality Chasm: A new health system for the 21st century*. Washington, DC: National Academies Press.

Jegers, M., Kesteloot, K., De Graeve, D. and Gilles, W. (2002) A typology for provider payment systems in health care, *Health Policy*, 60 (3): 255–73.

Lagarde, M. (2011) Provider payments, in L. Guinness and W. Wiseman (eds) *Introduction to Health Economics* (2nd edn). Maidenhead: Open University Press.

Langenbrunner, J., Orosz, E., Kutzin, J. and Wiley, M. (2005) Purchasing and paying providers, in J. Figueras, E. Jakubowski and R. Robinson (eds) *Purchasing to Improve Health Systems Performance*. Maidenhead: Open University Press.

Langenbrunner, J. and Wiley, C. (2002) Hospital payment mechanisms: theory and practice in transition countries, in M. McKee and J. Healy (eds) *Hospitals in a Changing Europe*. Buckingham: Open University Press.

Langdown, C. and Peckham, S. (2014) The use of financial incentives to help improve health outcomes: is the quality and outcomes framework fit for purpose? A systematic review, *Journal of Public Health (Oxford)*, 36 (2): 251–8.

McIntyre, D. (2007) *Learning from Experience: Health care financing in low- and middle-income countries*. Geneva: Global Forum for Health Research.

Rice, T. (2006) The physician as the patient's agent, in A.M. Jones (ed.) *The Elgar Companion to Health Economics*. Cheltenham: Elgar Publishing.

Ryan, A.M. (2009) Effects of the Premier Hospital Quality Incentive Demonstration on Medicare patient mortality and cost, *Health Services Research*, 44 (3): 821–42.

Schneider, P. (2008) Provider payment reforms: lessons from Europe and the US for South Eastern Europe, in C. Bredenkamp, M. Gragnolati and V. Ramljak (eds) *Challenges and Reform Opportunities Facing Health and Pension Systems in the Western Balkans*. Washington, DC: International Bank for Reconstruction and Development/World Bank.

SECTION 4

Outcomes and quality of health care

SECTION 4

Outcomes and quality of health care

Quality of health services   10

This is the first of four chapters on managing the quality of health services. You have examined inputs and processes in earlier chapters but now you will look at how to measure the outcomes of health care – that is, the change (hopefully improvement) in the health of patients. In this chapter, you will learn what aspects of a patient's health should be measured, how they can be measured, and the characteristics of a good measure. In particular, you will learn about patient reported outcomes. In the following three chapters, you will consider how high quality can be defined, how the performance of health services can be assessed, and finally how practice and policy can be changed to improve quality.

Learning objectives

After working through this chapter, you will be able to:

• distinguish between inputs, processes, and outcomes
• define and describe the key dimensions of health that need to be measured (impairment, disability, and quality of life)
• appreciate the opportunities and challenges of using patient reported outcomes
• understand how to assess the quality of a measure

Key terms

Disability (functional status): The impact of an impairment on the patient's ability to function.

Health-related quality of life (handicap, well-being): The impact of disability (functional status) on a person's social functioning, partly determined by their environment and circumstances (e.g. housing, economic status).

Impairment: The physical signs of the condition (pathology), usually measured objectively by clinicians.

Patient experience: The patient's views of the humanity of the care they receive, covering such aspects as respect and dignity, receiving information, waiting times, etc. Seeks to be objective, avoiding patient's subjective expectations.

Patient reported outcome measures (PROMs): Outcomes reported by patients using questionnaires that may be generic (general aspects of a person's health, such as mobility, sleeping, and appetite) or disease-specific (focused on a particular disease). Also referred to as patient reported outcomes (PROs).

Patient satisfaction: Patients' satisfaction with the humanity of care received. Influenced by a patient's expectations.

Quality care: Care that is safe, effective, humane, equitable, and sustainable.

Quality management: A systematic approach to quality of care that encompasses defining, assessing, and improving the quality of health services.

Reliability: The extent to which an instrument (e.g. clinical test, questionnaire) produces consistent results.

Responsiveness: The extent to which an instrument (e.g. clinical test, questionnaire) detects real changes in the state of health of a person.

Sustainability: The capacity of health services/systems to endure financially, socially, and environmentally.

Validity: The extent to which an instrument (e.g. clinical test, questionnaire) measures what it intends to measure.

What is quality?

The principal aim for everyone involved in the management of health services, regardless of whether they are making policy, providing care, commissioning or regulating services, is to improve the quality of care with the resources available. 'Quality' and 'quality of care' are terms that are widely used in many articles and books you read. And you could be forgiven for being unsure what the authors mean, as quality is a term that is used rather vaguely.

✎ Activity 10.1

One simple way of understanding what the word 'quality' means is to define what you mean by a high quality health service. So, complete the sentence: 'A high quality health service would provide care that is . . .'

Feedback

'A high quality health service would provide care that is . . .'

- *safe* – does no harm
- *effective* – does good (patients benefit)
- *humane* – treats people with respect, in a timely fashion, gives them the information they want, etc.
- *equitable* – available to all who could benefit from it regardless of sex, age, ethnicity, etc.

Note that this definition does not include any consideration of the cost of care. That is because the key challenge for health care policy-makers and managers is to provide good quality care at a reasonable cost (ensuring the greatest benefit at least cost). It therefore makes no sense to include 'cost' within the definition of quality. 'Efficiency' and 'productivity' are laudable aims but they are indications of the relationship between quality and cost, not a dimension of quality.

It is also important to recognize that as resources are always limited, it is not possible to maximize all four dimensions of quality. For example, if you want to achieve high equity of access to care (e.g. everyone has a health centre within one kilometre of their home), it will not be possible to maximize effectiveness because highly expert care cannot be provided in all sites (as there would have to be health centres even in remote areas with just a few scattered homesteads). So, equity of access would only be achieved by sacrificing effectiveness (and thus also equity of outcomes). In other words, trade-offs have to be made, often referred to as 'hard choices'. This is why it should not be left entirely to experts to decide on the format of a health system but decisions must involve the public (or their representatives, such as politicians) who have to consider explicitly the value they put on each dimension of quality. In practice, politicians and the public find that it is easier to choose, usually reluctantly, which short-comings are acceptable (e.g. some lack of equity to ensure greater efficiency) than having to select the positive aspects they want (which understandably will end up including everything).

There is one other dimension of quality that has largely been neglected and only recently been recognized as important – that of sustainability. This is not traditionally included in considerations of quality but needs to be considered. Sustainability refers to the capacity of the health care system and services to endure financially, socially, and environmentally. Increasingly the focus is on the last of these. You need to consider the impact of health services on the environment – on carbon emissions, water requirements, air pollution.

Fortunately, some innovations to improve the established dimensions of quality may also reduce the environmental impact of services. For example, Bond and colleagues (2009) have shown that providing a mobile breast screening caravan in an English rural district led to fewer car journeys to a central hospital facility by women, saving 75 tons of carbon dioxide a year. However, as with the established dimensions of quality, there may be trade-offs. Zander and colleagues (2011) have shown that the introduction of primary angioplasty for acute myocardial infarctions (heart attacks) in place of using thrombolytic drugs required longer ambulance journeys (to take patients to more distant regional centres), leading to a 3.2-fold increase in carbon emissions.

 Activity 10.2

While studies evaluating specific interventions are important, David Pencheon (2013) argues for the need to think in radically different ways about how the challenges of providing health and social care are conceived and approached. As you read the following edited version of his editorial, identify the three key components he suggests for transforming the objectives, the values, and the incentives of health and social care.

Developing a sustainable health and care system: lessons for research and policy

Every health and care system faces an increasing range of challenges as it tries to improve quality within financial and environmental limits, while demand and the cost of technologies rise. However, it is unlikely that these challenges will be addressed successfully and sustainably unless they are considered, not as separate problems, but at a system level. In this context, sustainability means meeting current challenges without prejudicing the ability of those in the future to do the same. It also means understanding the close relationship and synergy between environmental sustainability, social justice, resilient people and communities, and financial sustainability. This involves taking the future as seriously as the present. The good news is that taking our future environment seriously can also deliver immediate health benefits.

Three challenges stand out. First, we need to understand not only the needs of a changing population (demographic, social, cultural) but also the assets and willingness of people to collaborate and take more control of their health and wellbeing, with appropriate support. Second, the rapid growth of science and technology has important implications for how a health and care system can improve efficiency. Third, public services need to act within environmental, as well as financial boundaries and under an increasing level of regulation and scrutiny. Health and care systems have both a responsibility and an opportunity to demonstrate a commitment to taking our future health seriously, as large employers, as large procurers and as leading exemplars of how large organizations should be behaving in the interests of our common future. Unless we develop a system-wide approach we may not succeed. Increasing the efficiency of the current system is necessary but not enough. We need to simultaneously reassess, realign and transform the objectives, the values and the incentives.

Three parts of this transition are particularly important. First, demographic changes mean building a more collaborative, localized and enabling approach to helping people live lives they have reason to value . . . The priority for all agencies should be, collaboratively, to create the best possible conditions locally where this can happen, and to complement this with high quality services with sustainability as one of the dimensions of quality. Preventable illness and unplanned hospital admissions should be seen as signs of system failure until proved otherwise. Financial and other incentives should be aligned accordingly between agencies, embedded within the system's values, regulations and rewards. This means more outcome-based reward systems, clearer partnerships and more mature commissioning arrangements. This transition mirrors the transition from a product to a service-based approach considered a hallmark of environmentally sustainable systems more generally . . .

Second, technology needs to be harnessed to help people live as close to home as possible and to personalize preventive care and support systems . . . A clearer understanding of risk (using genomic analysis and risk stratification) and a better appreciation of personal preferences could improve the targeting and efficiency of health care and social support. The default place for care is the home and the default carer is the person with their family and friends, with the support of more formal services in the home and other settings. Technology should create the right conditions for people and communities to take much more control of their own health. Understanding how we use nineteenth-century inventions such as the telephone in the 21st century would be a welcome advance for the health and care system. It is good value, convenient, promotes better access and is environmentally appropriate.

Third, the challenge of operating within environmental limits (as well as financial and legal limits) should accelerate accountability, openness and innovation and should stimulate a culture where the genuine involvement of users can help shape better models of care. Increasing health care spending brings smaller marginal gains in health and sometimes may even be associated with poorer health outcomes . . .

The evidence suggests we can combine some of the individual challenges we face, into a set of interrelated solutions that are fundamental to sustainable, affordable and fairer systems of health and care. If so, we can improve our health today in ways that do not disproportionately harm the health of others elsewhere or in future. We have neither the right to knowingly perpetuate global and intergenerational inequities, nor do we have the need to do so when so many health co-benefits are associated with action now. The research and policy agenda should focus on understanding how we implement the evidence we already have to shape the policies we need. Future generations might not forgive us for knowing so much and doing so little. (Pencheon, 2013)

Feedback

The three key components of transforming the objectives, the values, and the incentives of health and social care suggested are:

1 Building a more collaborative, localized, and enabling approach to helping people live lives they have reason to value.
2 Harnessing technology to help people remain as close to home as possible and to personalize preventive care and support systems.
3 Operating within environmental limits so as to accelerate accountability, openness, and innovation.

Structure, processes, and outcomes

To assess and improve the quality of health services, it is necessary to be able to measure each dimension in rigorous ways. In 1966, Avedis Donabedian, a physician and health services researcher at the University of Michigan, proposed a model that provides a framework for assessing the quality of health care (Donabedian, 2003). He suggested that information about quality can be drawn from three categories: structure, processes, and outcomes. *Structure* describes the inputs to care including buildings, staff, finance, and equipment. *Processes* are the transactions between patients and providers throughout the delivery of care (such as a treatment). *Outcomes* are the effects of care on the health of patients and populations. While there are other quality of care frameworks, including the WHO Quality of Care Framework and the Bamako Initiative, Donabedian's model continues to dominate and has the advantage of being simple and elegant.

Ultimately, what the public are concerned about is outcomes – are you more or less likely to survive or get better with one provider or practitioner rather than another? However, measurement and collection of data on outcomes are usually complex and expensive. At the other extreme, inputs can be measured cheaply and easily but may not provide a valid indication of performance. For example, for safety it will be much easier to measure the number of doctors per 1000 patients than to measure an outcome such as the number of missed diagnoses or surgical errors. However, the former is only a valid indication of safety if there is good scientific evidence that more doctors per 1000 patients is associated with safer care.

In the middle are process measures that are easier to collect than outcomes and do not involve any delay in waiting to determine the patient's outcome, which may not be clear for months or years. While process measures are often the best option, as with inputs, they are only valid if they are associated with good outcomes. For example, it is widely recognized that people who have suffered a heart attack are more likely to survive if they are treated with thrombolytic drugs (which prevent blood clotting). It is, therefore, valid to assess the effectiveness of health services for people suffering a heart attack by measuring the proportion who receive this drug promptly. In contrast, many countries use the rate of patient readmissions to hospital as a measure of safety and/or effectiveness of care. This assumes that the readmission rate is a valid indication of safety or effectiveness of care. However, there is no or little association with valid outcome measures, a finding that should not surprise you given that, as you saw in Chapter 7, admission rates depend to a large extent on clinicians' judgements.

In contrast to inputs and processes, measuring outcomes is much more challenging, as it requires us to measure a person's state of health. This requires us to address four questions:

- What aspect of a person's health should be measured?
- How can health be measured?
- What is a good measure?
- Which measure to use?

What aspect of a person's health should be measured?

This depends on what impact you expect the intervention to have. For example, if you expect the death rate from the condition to be reduced, it would be reasonable to consider mortality as an outcome. But mortality would be inappropriate if the intervention has little impact on survival but instead aims to improve a patient's mobility or lessen their symptoms (e.g. treatment of arthritis).

There are five aspects of health status to choose from when selecting appropriate outcomes to measure:

- Death/survival
- Impairment – the physical signs of the condition (pathology) usually measured objectively by clinicians
- Symptoms – reported by the patient
- Disability (also referred to as functional status) – the impact on the patient's ability to function (e.g. mobility)
- Health-related quality of life (also referred to as handicap and wellbeing) – the impact of the condition on the social functioning of a person, partly determined by a person's environment

Apart from mortality, the other four are related to one another. This can be seen best if you consider an example. A common problem among elderly men is that their prostate enlarges, causing several urinary symptoms such as having to urinate more frequently, including during the night, thus disturbing their sleep. Figure 10.1 illustrates the relationship between the four aspects of health status and whether they are reported by a clinician or the patient.

Impairment refers to the effect the condition has on their physiology. In this case, because there is partial obstruction at the neck of the bladder, the rate at which a man can urinate is reduced (referred to as the urine flow rate). This can be detected by a clinician but it is not the reason that men present to their doctor.

What they actually complain about are the symptoms (pain on passing urine) and the effect the condition is having on their functioning, such as having to go to the toilet frequently.

This needs to be distinguished from the fourth aspect, the impact that the condition has on a person's quality of life. How bothersome the disability is will vary between patients and depend to a considerable extent on the physical, social, and psychological environment. If a man is a train driver and cannot easily leave the train cab to go to the toilet frequently, the

Reported by:	Aspects of health status			
	Symptoms	Impairment	Disability/functional status	Health-related quality of life
Patient	Pain on passing urine		Having to go to the toilet frequently	Unable to sit through film in cinema
Clinician		Reduced urine flow rate		

Figure 10.1 Aspects of health status using the example of benign prostatic hyperplasia

condition will have a major impact because he may be unable to continue in his job. In contrast, going to the toilet frequently may be nothing more than a nuisance for an office worker.

 Activity 10.3

How could the health of someone with arthritis of the hip be assessed? You need to consider their impairment, symptoms, disability, and quality of life.

Feedback

You should have identified the following:

- Impairment could be assessed by a clinician examining the extent to which the person can move their leg, or X-ray findings.
- Symptoms could be assessed by administering a standard pain questionnaire.
- Disability could be assessed in terms of how far they can walk without pain.
- Quality of life could be assessed in terms of the impact their disability is having on the activities they like to do (e.g. gardening, playing sports, shopping).

While these four aspects are related to one another, it is not a straightforward relationship. The extent to which someone is disabled can be explained to some extent by the level of impairment. But research shows that only about 50 per cent of a person's disability is 'explained' by their impairment. This is because people have considerable capacity to compensate and learn to accommodate their impairment. People learn ways of coping with impairment – the Para-Olympics is a shining example of how far some people can go to overcome impairment.

Similarly, disability does not automatically affect a person's quality of life. Only about 50 per cent of a person's quality of life is explained by their level of disability. So, the man who has to visit the toilet every hour but loves going to the cinema will ensure he sits at the end of a row so he doesn't disturb others. Quality of life is affected by many things (such as housing, employment, relationships) not just a person's health. So it is not surprising that impairment has only a partial influence (50% × 50% = 25%) on quality of life. This is why it is necessary to restrict considerations to people's quality of life to what is defined as their 'health-related quality of life' when measuring the impact of health care.

How can a person's health be measured?

The measurement of mortality is obvious and usually straightforward, although in high-income countries in recent years there have been debates about how death is defined – the moment at which the heart and lungs stop functioning or when the brain stops functioning? The development of life-support technology that can maintain a person's breathing has raised medical and ethical questions about the distinction between dead and alive.

As you have seen in Figure 10.1, measurement of the four other aspects of health requires a mixture of clinician and patient involvement:

- *Impairment* is assessed by a clinician and involves objective observation and measurement. It may focus on such things as the person's physiology, biochemistry or immune status. Measurement may be quite simple such as weighing scales and a tape measure to determine how well a child is growing, although increasingly, particularly in high-income countries, it involves expensive high-tech equipment such as scanners.
- *Symptoms* can only be reported by patients, as they generally cannot be observed by clinicians. They can be measured using validated questionnaires to determine features such as their frequency and severity.
- In contrast, *disability* may be assessed by clinicians or patients. For example, the distance a patient can walk, or the weight a person can lift, can be assessed by either the patient or the clinician.
- *Health-related quality of life* is, by definition, a subjective assessment of how a person's state of health is affecting them socially and psychologically. The only person who can assess this is the person him or herself. You may have a view of the quality of someone else's life but that may differ markedly from that person's self-assessment. For example, able-bodied observers may feel that someone requiring a wheelchair has a poor quality of life but that may not be the view of the affected person.

There is now widespread recognition of the need for patients to assess key aspects of their health: symptoms, functional status, health-related quality of life. The questionnaires (also referred to as instruments) used to do this are known as Patient Reported Outcomes (PROs) or Patient Reported Outcome Measures (PROMs).

Which patient reported outcome measure to use?

A key consideration is between *generic* and *disease-specific measures.* Generic measures, as the term implies, measure general aspects of health rather than those aspects that are affected by a particular disease.

The most widely used generic measures are the EuroQuol (EQ-5D), which has five questions (or items), and the Short Form 36 (SF36), which contains 36 questions. The latter covers eight domains:

- Physical functioning
- Role physical
- Bodily pain
- General health perception
- Energy/vitality
- Social functioning
- Role emotional
- Mental health.

The advantage of using a generic, rather than disease-specific, measure is that you can then compare the benefit that patients with disease X gain from treatment with the benefit gained by patients with disease Y. The disadvantage is that because it is generic, several domains being measured may not be relevant to people with the disease or treatment being assessed. As a result, generic measures will not be as sensitive in detecting and quantifying the effect of an intervention as a disease-specific measure. For example, a measure for assessing hip replacement surgery would focus on the amount of hip pain and mobility – the two principal aspects for which you should see an improvement. The advantage is that disease-specific measures are highly responsive. The disadvantage is that you cannot compare the benefits of hip surgery with that of, say, malaria treatment.

Another consideration is whether you measure the *final outcome* or an *intermediate outcome*. The final outcome is what you are trying to achieve by intervening. For example, treatment for diabetes aims to prevent long-term consequences such as blindness or kidney disease. Therefore, to assess using the final outcome, you would need to wait many years. However, governments, health services, and the public might want to know what effect the programme is having much sooner than that. What you could do is use an intermediate outcome, such as the frequency of hyperglycaemic attacks.

Many generic and disease-specific measures have been developed and lists of those available can be found online. When choosing which to use, you should ensure that its validity and reliability have been rigorously tested and shown to be good.

- *Validity* – does the instrument measure what it intends to measure?
- *Reliability* – does the instrument produce consistent results?

For example, when weighing babies in a child health clinic, validity relates to whether weight is an indicator of a baby's health and reliability relates to whether the weight recorded would be the same if repeated. There are two ways in which the reliability can be tested. If two or more people use the measure, do they get the same answer? This is as important a consideration for doctors interpreting an X-ray (do they all see the same things?) as it is for two people interviewing a patient about their quality of life. This is known as *inter-observer* (or *inter-rater*) *reliability*. You also want to know that if a measure is used again by the same observer, you will get the same answer (assuming the patient's health has not altered between the two assessments). This is known *as intra-observer reliability*.

Finally, you need to consider when to assess the impact of a health care intervention. For practical reasons, you want to know about the outcome as soon as possible (e.g. when assessing the effectiveness of a hospital) but too short an observation period may render misleading results if all the benefits have not yet become apparent (e.g. it may take up to a year to see the benefits of a knee joint replacement).

Two potential misunderstandings

With increasing acceptance of the importance of collecting and using patients' reports to determine the quality of health care, it is important to avoid two common misunderstandings. The first is the distinction between patients' reports of the effectiveness (or outcome) of care and their experience of care. You have learnt how patients can report on the effectiveness of care using PROMs. But patients can also play a key role in measuring another dimension of quality, that of the humanity of care. Patients' experience of the processes of care (such as, were they treated with dignity and respect?, were they kept waiting?, etc.) can also be collected using patient reported experience measures (PREMs).

Activity 10.4

In the following edited account by Nick Black and Crispin Jenkinson (2009), they consider the challenge of using patients' reports to assess the quality of services. As you read it, consider the following questions:

1 What are some of the challenges to using PROMs in areas of care other than elective surgery?
2 Why has the emphasis shifted from assessing patients' satisfaction with care to their experience of care?

Measuring patients' experiences and outcomes

There is now a widespread realisation that patients' views are not optional but essential to achieving high quality care . . . Patients offer a complementary perspective to that of clinicians, providing unique information and insights into both the humanity of care (such as dignity and respect, privacy, meeting information needs, waiting and delays, and cleanliness of facilities) and the effectiveness of health care . . . Greater recognition and acceptance of the contribution of patients over the past two decades have been accompanied and facilitated by a major growth in the development of rigorous instruments (questionnaires) . . .

Concern has shifted from measuring patients' satisfaction with the humanity of care to measuring their experience of the humanity of care (that is, seeking value-free reports of cleanliness, dignity, etc.). This is because the measures of satisfaction were strongly influenced by patients' expectations, which could be quite low, and were found to be fairly insensitive in detecting shortcomings . . .

Although clinicians can make objective observations of signs, impairment, and disability, only patients can report on their symptoms and quality of life. Many instruments exist for reporting these aspects. Most are specific for a condition or procedure. For example, the Oxford hip score for patients with hip osteoarthrosis and the international prostate symptom score for patients with benign prostate disease. Although referred to in the UK as patient reported outcome measures (PROMs), they are actually measures of health status; the outcome of care has to be derived by comparing data collected at different times (for example, before and after surgery). There are also some generic instruments (such as the EQ-5D and the SF-36) that are designed to be used with any patients. These are less sensitive than disease-specific instruments but allow comparisons between patients with different conditions . . .

Directories and systematic reviews of available instruments exist to help select the most appropriate one. The better directories provide independent assessment of the validity, reliability, responsiveness, and feasibility (cost, time to complete, acceptability) of instruments. But that is not sufficient; instruments must be used rigorously to ensure confidence in the findings: are the patients representative? Are sufficient numbers included? Is there recruitment bias? Are the outcomes measured at the appropriate time after an intervention? . . .

Current enthusiasm for involving patients in measuring the humanity and effectiveness of care should not obscure the challenges . . . The best time to request patients' views is not always obvious. Generally speaking, views on the humanity of care need to be assessed fairly soon after using a service to prevent recall bias . . . Some delay is needed when obtaining patients' views of outcomes to ensure all potential benefits have been realised . . .

The effectiveness of elective surgery is relatively straightforward to assess, as patients have a discrete intervention and their health status can be assessed before and after, but long-term conditions, such as diabetes, require assessments at regular intervals (perhaps six-monthly) and the goal may be to maintain, or avoid deterioration in, health status rather than a significant improvement. Acute emergencies represent another challenge as it is impossible to obtain the pre-event health status of patients (except by recall, which is of uncertain validity). One option is to compare the patient's report of their health status once they have recovered from the acute episode with age-sex standardised population norms.

Patients who are unable to self-report because of physical or mental impairment present another challenge. One option is to rely on their lay carers (relatives, friends) to act as proxy respondents. Clearly, the danger is that the reported views partly depend on the proxy's observation and interpretation . . .

There is the challenge of reconciling patients' and clinicians' reports of outcomes . . . what if clinicians report an improvement in impairment (such as a better urine flow rate after prostate surgery) but patients report no improvement in their symptoms (still experiencing nocturia four times a night)? This raises the question of the relative importance of the different dimensions of health (impairment, symptoms, disability, quality of life, complications), the answer depending on the perspective of the questioner.

Traditionally, the person at the centre of health care had no real voice. Professionals judged the quality of services. Now, the patient is central in the hope this will contribute to quality improvement . . . The benefits of such changes could revolutionise how health care is evaluated. Patient reporting is not a panacea, but considering patients' views in a systematic and thoughtful manner is a first step to incorporating them into clinical practice.

From Black, N. and Jenkinson, C. (2009) How can patients' views of their care enhance quality improvement?, *British Medical Journal*, 339: 202–5, with permission from BMJ Publishing Group Ltd.

Feedback

1   Some of the challenges to using PROMs more widely are:

   • Unlike elective surgery, long-term conditions do not have a 'before and after' or a cure.
   • It's not possible to collect data before an emergency condition.
   • Some patients are not able to report (e.g. those with severe dementia).

2   Measures of satisfaction with the humanity of care are strongly influenced by patients' expectations, whereas measures of experience attempt to obtain less subjective accounts.

This introduces the second potential cause of confusion in the field of measurement that you need to be aware of: the distinction between subjective and objective measures. This distinction is often confused with whether or not the measurement can be 'trusted'. People often assume that objective measures are 'better' than subjective ones. This is incorrect.

✏ Activity 10.5

This issue is addressed in the following edited essay by Paul Cleary (1997), an expert in health status measurement. As you read it, make notes on why subjective measures should be included when assessing people's health state.

Subjective and objective measures of health: which is better when?

Clinicians and biomedical researchers frequently question the value of subjective measures of health. Whether a measure is subjective (based on individual awareness or experience) or objective (existing and measurable, independent of individual experiences) certainly is an important characteristic of variables related to health states. However, it is my experience that participants in such debates often confuse the distinction between variable type and measurement strategy. For example, some researchers are uncomfortable with the results of surveys about health-related quality of life and would prefer to use only data derived from medical record reviews for their analyses. It is important to understand both the inherent characteristics of the variables we are interested in and the strengths and weaknesses of different measurement strategies if we are to obtain the best possible data for health and health services studies . . .

Which aspects of health should be measured depends on the hypotheses being tested. For example, if the hypothesis is that a particular dietary supplement will increase the number of red cells in the blood, then measures of symptoms, difficulty performing basic activities of daily living, or general health perceptions are probably not needed . . . If, however, one wants to assess the impact of improving the red cell concentration on patients' lives, it would be important to measure aspects of health-related quality of life . . .

Subjective measures can sometimes also provide accurate and efficient assessments of objective states. Physical functioning is such a variable. Patients can be asked whether they have difficulty going up and down stairs, or an observer can visit their homes to observe whether they can or cannot climb stairs. This is a situation in which objective measures are available and can be more reliable and valid, if properly administered, than patient self-reports, but such methods are often prohibitively expensive. Extensive research in this area has led to the development of short, functional status measures that can be administered directly to patients very efficiently and which have excellent reliability and validity. Thus, the use of such subjective measures is now widely accepted.

Probably the most subjective concept in health status assessment is perceived health. A typical question used to assess this variable is: 'Overall, how would you rate your health?' Respondents usually are then provided with a five-point Likert scale (poor, good, very good, excellent) or a 0–10 rating scale on which they can rate their health. To those trained in physical or biological sciences, this type of measure may seem problematic. What exactly does this variable measure? How can one possibly interpret such a subjective impression?

This measure is known to mean different things to different people and, in some ways, that is its strength. We view general health perception as an individual's synthesis of various objective and subjective information about health that integrates this information using individual weights and preferences. Whether this is a good thing to measure is partly a matter of opinion, but it is also an empirical issue ... The empirical question is whether such a measure provides information that other variables do not, and/or whether it reliably predicts phenomena of interest.

One of the most compelling reasons for assessing general perceived health is that it predicts subsequent morbidity and mortality, even after controlling for other biological and health status variables. For example, self-evaluations of health predict mortality, even after statistically controlling for the presence of health problems, disability, and/or other risk factors. It has been found that elderly people with perceived poor health were six times as likely to die in a 4-year period than those who reported that their health was excellent – a relative risk greater than that for smoking (Idler and Kasl, 1991).

We do not fully understand why perceived health is such a good predictor of mortality. There may be other unmeasured objective measures of health that could reduce the residual explanatory predictive power of perceived health. However, considering the sophistication of available studies, the power of this variable is striking. Several reasons why this variable predicts mortality have been posited. It may reflect a self-fulfilling prophesy. That is, people who think they are in poor health may not protect and promote their health as much as other people. Another explanation is that such ratings may capture more information than is available in other types of assessments. When individuals rate their health, they may consider family, genetic and health history information, information about their physical and social environment, and their own attitudes and expectations about health, in addition to numerous signs and symptoms related to their health. People may use their knowledge and experience to provide a more integrated and informative rating than is possible with other variables typically available to researchers. Irrespective of which explanation is correct, data on the relationships between mortality rates and subjective states such as chest pain or general health perception should put to rest any qualms about the value of subjective measures of health.

Some researchers are uncomfortable with subjective variables because they are perceived as unreliable. Such people often think of data from medical records as 'hard' data, whereas they think of survey responses as 'soft' data'. Thus, rather than judging the relative theoretical value of objective and subjective measures, some researchers' selection of variables is unduly influenced by their negative opinions about the value of survey data relative to other types of information . . .

Even though symptoms are inherently subjective, some researchers seem to feel more comfortable using medical record notations, rather than information from patient surveys, as symptom measures. However, a measure of chest pain collected using a standardized instrument, such as the Rose questionnaire, using rigorous sampling and survey administration techniques, will yield a measure that is more reliable and valid than indications in medical records that were collected using different techniques by many clinicians who had their own subjective impressions of how 'sick' an individual patient was.

Many 'objective' or partly objective variables, such as functional status, probably are best measured using objective methods. However, it is important to recognize that abstracting such information from medical records does not mean that it is 'objective'. Medical records frequently contain functional assessments that were obtained by health care professionals with no training in standardized measurement and that are largely subjective measures. Such variables may be measured more efficiently, reliably and validly with standardized subjective measures.

Many clinical, health services and health policy studies test hypotheses based on subjective variables. We need to learn a great deal more about individual variations in how people perceive, interpret and report subjective states such as symptoms and general health perception. Nevertheless, concern about reliability and validity, although always an over-riding research consideration, should not preclude considerations of subjective variables since extensive methodological research on the measurement of such variables has led to techniques that allow researchers to measure them with a level of reliability and validity that frequently exceeds the assessment of objective states. The types of variables to be assessed in any given study should be determined on the basis of the hypotheses being tested, not on poorly founded opinions about the value of different data collection strategies.

Reproduced from Cleary (1997). With permission of the Royal Society of Medicine Press Limited.

Feedback

Subjective measures may:

- be the appropriate aspect to be assessed, e.g. if the treatment is intended to improve a patient's quality of life;
- provide a more efficient means of assessing an objective state, e.g. a mailed self-completed questionnaire is a cheaper way of ascertaining how far someone can walk than sending an observer to visit them;

- provide more valid assessment of a person's health state and prognosis;
- provide a more reliable assessment, as new data using standard definitions may be used whereas 'objective' data in medical records is dependent on the definitions used by each and every clinician recording the information.

Managing quality

Having learnt about the dimensions of quality and about different aspects of outcome and how to measure them, we now consider the three stages of how we can manage the quality of care provided (Figure 10.2).

Having selected a topic, either clinical (such as a particular treatment) or organizational (such as how to deliver care), the first stage is to *define good quality* in terms of criteria and standards. How this is done will be addressed in Chapter 11. It is then necessary to *assess the quality of care* actually being provided, considered in Chapter 12. And finally, and the hardest stage, it is necessary to take action to *improve quality*. The relationship between these three stages can be presented in the form of a cycle, shown in Figure 10.2. The reason to show it as a cycle rather than just a simple linear model is because it is necessary to re-assess quality, having intervened to improve it, to make sure the desired improvements have occurred. If they haven't, which is often the case, it will be necessary

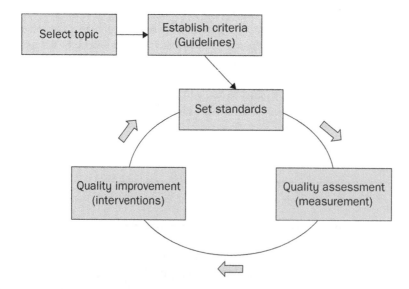

Figure 10.2 Quality management cycle

to intervene again, perhaps in a different way, and once again assess quality to ensure improvements have occurred.

Summary

People's state of health can be assessed in terms of symptoms, impairment, disability, and health-related quality of life. Any measure, whether subjective or objective, must be valid, reliable, and responsive. Consistent with a shift towards more patient-centred care, it is important to include patients' reports of the effectiveness and humanity of their care. This will involve considering whether or not to use generic or disease-specific measures, or both. Many such measures have been developed and ones that have been properly tested and evaluated should be selected. Devising a new measure is a complex, time-consuming process and should only be considered if no suitable measure exists.

References

Black, N. and Jenkinson, C. (2009) How can patients' views of their care enhance quality improvement?, *British Medical Journal*, 339: 202–5.

Bond, A., Jones, A., Haynes, R., Tam, M., Denton, E., Ballantyne, M. et al. (2009) Tackling climate change close to home: mobile breast screening as a mode, *Journal of Health Services Research and Policy*, 14 (3): 165–7.

Cleary, P.D. (1997) Subjective and objective measures of health: which is better when?, *Journal of Health Services Research and Policy*, 2 (1): 3–4.

Donabedian, A. (2003) *An Introduction to Quality Assurance in Health Care* (Vol. 1). New York: Oxford University Press.

Idler, E.L. and Kasl, S. (1991) Health perceptions and survival: do global evaluations of health status really predict mortality?, *Journal of Gerontology*, 46 (2): S55–65.

Pencheon, D. (2013) Developing a sustainable health and care system: lessons for research and policy, *Journal of Health Services Research and Policy*, 18 (4): 193–4.

Zander, A., Niggebrugge, A., Pencheon, D. and Lyratazopoulis, G. (2011) Changes in travel-related carbon emissions associated with modernization of services for patients with acute myocardial infarction: a case study, *Journal of Public Health*, 33 (2): 272–9.

11 Defining good quality health services

Overview

This is the second of four chapters on managing the quality of health services. This chapter focuses on the first step – that of defining what constitutes good quality. You will learn of the importance of trust and professional accountability, about how the available research evidence should be used, and then how it can be combined with professional experience, using consensus development methods, to create guidelines. The following two chapters will consider how, using definitions of good quality care, the performance of health services can be assessed and finally how practice and policy can be improved.

Learning objectives

After working through this chapter, you will be able to:

- explain why formal means for defining high quality care are needed to ensure professionals are accountable to the public
- describe what evidence-based medicine is
- explain why policy is influenced but not necessarily based on scientific evidence
- describe how research evidence can be reviewed systematically
- describe how consensus development methods can be used to develop clinical guidelines

Key terms

Clinical guidelines: Advice based on the best available research evidence and the consensus view of clinicians.

Consensus development: A set of explicit formal methods for developing and establishing the collective views of a group when faced with uncertainty.

Evidence-based medicine: The conscientious, explicit, and judicious use of current best evidence in making decisions about the care of individual patients.

Public trust: The expectation that professionals will be knowledgeable and competent and will behave in the patient's best interest with beneficence, fairness, and integrity.

Systematic review: A review of the literature that uses an explicit approach to searching, selecting, and combining the relevant studies.

Trust and accountability

Before considering how the quality of health services can be managed, it is important to pause and consider why it is felt necessary to invest so many resources in defining, assessing, and improving the quality of health care. In essence, it is because the public cannot assume that all is well just because health care professionals say so. In other words, the public and patients cannot automatically trust professionals.

Activity 11.1

There is evidence that the level of public trust has fallen over recent years in high-income countries, a view held by Huw Davies (1999) in the following edited article. As you read it, consider the following questions:

1 What does the author mean by 'public trust'?
2 How can accountability be achieved?

Falling public trust in health services: implications for accountability

What is public trust? In the literature, definitions differ but all embody the notion of expectations: expectations by the public that health care providers will demonstrate knowledge, skill and competence; further expectations too that they will behave as true agents (that is, in the patient's best interest) and with beneficence, fairness and integrity. It is these collective expectations that form the basis of trust, and these same expectations that can be shaken by repeated demonstrations that all is not well with health care. Trust is slowly gained but easily lost in the face of confounded expectations.

We should not underestimate the potential importance of falling public trust in health services. Although unfounded trust is merely hope and dependency (and its loss may be no loss at all), a robust public trust may be advantageous in many ways . . . Without trust we may have to turn to new ways of defining relationships. These new ways of managing relationships may in turn have further impact on trust. One of the key relationships on which public trust may have impact is the 'accountability relationship' between the public and various health care organizations.

*The public have a right to expect that health care organisations will oper-
ate effectively. To some extent, and this varies between countries, such
expectations are taken on trust. However, when trust is damaged, the
public seeks new routes to accountability . . .*

*Accountability can be achieved by a number of different routes. First,
organisations can provide formal accounts (such as annual reports) of
their mission, objectives, activities and progress. Such accounts may,
however, be seen as mainly 'public relations', putting a good gloss on
things and serving a largely ceremonial role. Thus, in health care, these
general accounts are increasingly supplemented by the publication of
specific performance data on a wide range of dimensions.*

*. . . Each approach to accountability has its own area of application, and
its own advantages, costs and burdens. With all the approaches there is
scope for perverse incentives and dysfunctional consequences (undesir-
able changes in behaviour in response to the accountability system). In
addition, there is some concern that changing emphases on external
accountability might exert influence on mechanisms of governance within
organisations in less than desirable ways. Most developed nations use an
ever-shifting mix of these different systems, as an over-reliance on any
single approach tends merely to highlight its flaws. Further, the routine
application of many of the approaches to accountability may lead to ritu-
alistic rather than instrumental systems.*

*. . . Before trust as a basis for the relationship between the public and
their health care services is further undermined, we should begin to identify how public trust sustains well-functioning organisations – especially
those agencies in the public sector that lack market discipline.*

*We also need a much clearer idea of whether and how too much trust
shields the incompetent. Finally, we still have only the vaguest ideas about
what nurtures public trust in the first place or impacts adversely upon it.
The role of the media may be crucial here, but this and other factors –
such as the rise of the consumer and the decline of the professional –
need to be examined both theoretically and empirically. . .*

Reproduced from Davies (1999). With permission of the Royal Society of Medicine
Press Limited.

Feedback

1   'Public trust' embodies the notion of the expectations the public have
    that clinicians will be knowledgeable, skilful, and competent; that they
    will behave in the patient's best interest with beneficence, fairness,
    and integrity.
2   Accountability can be achieved through formal accounts (e.g. annual
    reports) and the publication of performance data, backed up by
    methods of regulation such as accreditation. (You will learn more
    about such methods in Chapter 12.)

Evidence-based medicine

So how can high quality be defined? Some dimensions of quality can be defined simply on the basis of societal values and morals. This is true for the humanity of care (treating people the way you would want to be treated), for equity (treating people the same regardless of their demographic and socio-economic characteristics), and for safety (avoiding all harm to patients). In contrast, defining what care should be provided to achieve high quality as regards effectiveness requires scientific research evidence.

The approach to defining effective care is through the creation of guidelines. These are criteria (or statements) that aim to make explicit the best way to manage a patient or organize a service to ensure the likeliest possibility that there will be a good outcome. Inevitably, health care is not quite as simple as other activities such as cooking, where a recipe can provide reliable guidelines to follow (though even in that example the outcome will depend to some extent on the cook). The strengths and limitations of an explicit approach based on scientific evidence have been recognized by its proponents.

✎ Activity 11.2

The following is an edited version of a key editorial published in the *British Medical Journal* in 1996 written by some of the leading proponents of what became known as 'evidence based medicine (EBM)' (Sackett et al., 1996). It was published a few years after the concept of EBM had been introduced in an attempt to rebut critics and to clarify its role and purpose. As you read it, identify the key tension that the authors are addressing.

Evidence based medicine: what it is and what it isn't

Evidence based medicine is the conscientious, explicit, and judicious use of current best evidence in making decisions about the care of individual patients. The practice of evidence based medicine means integrating individual clinical expertise with the best available external clinical evidence from systematic research. By individual clinical expertise we mean the proficiency and judgment that individual clinicians acquire through clinical experience and clinical practice. Increased expertise is reflected in many ways, but especially in more effective and efficient diagnosis and in the more thoughtful identification and compassionate use of individual patients' predicaments, rights, and preferences in making clinical decisions about their care. By best available external clinical evidence we mean clinically relevant research, often from the basic sciences of medicine, but especially from patient-centred clinical research into the accuracy and precision of diagnostic tests (including the clinical examination), the power of prognostic markers, and the efficacy and safety of therapeutic, rehabilitative, and preventive regimens. External clinical evidence both invalidates previously accepted diagnostic tests and treatments and replaces them with new ones that are more powerful, more accurate, more efficacious, and safer.

Good doctors use both individual clinical expertise and the best available external evidence, and neither alone is enough. Without clinical expertise, practice risks becoming tyrannised by evidence, for even excellent external evidence may be inapplicable to or inappropriate for an individual patient. Without current best evidence, practice risks becoming rapidly out of date, to the detriment of patients.

This description of what evidence based medicine is helps clarify what evidence based medicine is not. Evidence based medicine is neither old hat nor impossible to practise. The argument that 'everyone already is doing it' falls before evidence of striking variations in both the integration of patient values into our clinical behaviour and in the rates with which clinicians provide interventions to their patients. The difficulties that clinicians face in keeping abreast of all the medical advances reported in primary journals are obvious from a comparison of the time required for reading (for general medicine, enough to examine 19 articles per day, 365 days per year) with the time available (well under an hour a week by British medical consultants, even on self-reports) . . .

Evidence based medicine is not 'cookbook' medicine. Because it requires a bottom-up approach that integrates the best external evidence with individual clinical expertise and patients' choice, it cannot result in slavish, cookbook approaches to individual patient care. External clinical evidence can inform, but can never replace, individual clinical expertise, and it is this expertise that decides whether the external evidence applies to the individual patient at all and, if so, how it should be integrated into a clinical decision. Similarly, any external guideline must be integrated with individual clinical expertise in deciding whether and how it matches the patient's clinical state, predicament, and preferences, and thus whether it should be applied. Clinicians who fear top-down cookbooks will find the advocates of evidence based medicine joining them at the barricades.

Some fear that evidence based medicine will be hijacked by purchasers and managers to cut the costs of health care. This would not only be a misuse of evidence based medicine but suggests a fundamental misunderstanding of its financial consequences. Doctors practising evidence based medicine will identify and apply the most efficacious interventions to maximise the quality and quantity of life for individual patients; this may raise rather than lower the cost of their care . . .

From Sackett, D.L. et al. (1996) Evidence based medicine: what it is and what it isn't, *British Medical Journal*, 312 (7023): 71–2, with permission from BMJ Publishing Group Ltd.

Feedback

The key tension that the authors are addressing is that between scientific evidence, which, inevitably, provides statistical probabilities as to what is likely to be the best medicine for a particular patient and the wisdom of a doctor based on all the anecdotal experiences they have accumulated. The authors advocate a balance between the two. In addition, they recognize that patients will differ in their preferences and the values they attach to different potential outcomes (e.g. the balance between a reduction in symptoms and the risk of an adverse side-effect).

Evidence-based policy-making?

Before considering how scientific evidence is used to define quality by way of creating guidelines, it is worth considering one impact of evidence-based medicine that has not been fully resolved over the past two decades. The emergence of evidence-based medicine in the early 1990s led some clinicians to challenge managers and policy-makers to be equally evidence-based. They argued that if doctors were expected to base their decisions on the findings of research, policy-makers and managers ought to as well. It seemed difficult to argue with the idea that scientific research should drive policy. However, it was based on an implied model that does not take into account the complexity of policy-making. There are several reasons why research evidence may have limited influence on policies. Unlike clinical practice:

- Policy-makers have to consider multiple factors, which include social, financial, strategic, terms and conditions of employees, and electoral considerations.
- Research evidence may legitimately be seen as irrelevant because it comes from a different sector or specialty, practice depends on tacit knowledge, or it is not applicable locally.
- There is less likelihood of a consensus about research evidence, given its greater complexity, scientific controversy, and different interpretations that can be made.
- Policy-makers have to contend with and consider other types of competing evidence such as personal experience and local circumstances.

In addition, policy-makers working at a national level and those managing local services such as a hospital, have to contend with other legitimate interests aside from scientific evidence. Figure 11.1 shows the principal forces at work, the importance of each depending on the country and

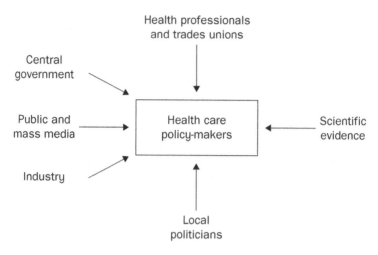

Figure 11.1 The environmental turbulence experienced by policy-makers

prevailing political, social, and cultural circumstances. This model demonstrates the turbulent environment in which policy-makers work, buffeted from all sides by different interest groups.

For all these reasons, the notion of evidence-based policy or evidence-based management should be considered cautiously. While scientific evidence has an important contribution to make, it is only one of many legitimate influences on policy-making. 'Evidence-influenced policy' is a more realistic aim for those advocating a greater role for scientific research. In contrast, guidance for much medical practice can be based on scientific evidence.

Creating guidelines

Preparation

Before embarking on creating a new guideline, it is sensible to determine whether one already exists. There are thousands of guidelines in existence and the number is increasing rapidly throughout the world. Two of the original organizations for creating guidelines were the Agency for Health Research & Quality (ARHQ) in the USA, which runs the National Guideline Clearinghouse (www.guideline.gov) and the National Institute for Health & Clinical Excellence (NICE) in the UK, which runs the National Clinical Guideline Centre (www.ncgc.ac.uk). Both are members of the Guidelines International Network (www.g-i-n.net/gin), which has 96 organizations from 79 countries. By 2015, their website contained over 6400 guidelines from around the world. Member organizations include international agencies, governments, health insurance companies, and professional associations.

✎ Activity 11.3

Can you suggest what criteria you would use to decide whether an existing guideline is suitable for your purposes?

Feedback

The sorts of issues you might have considered include:

- Is it up-to-date? Research evidence accumulates rapidly in some fields.
- Is it relevant to my country? Guidelines have to be relevant to the context in which they are going to be adopted, such as the level of health care expenditure or religious beliefs.
- Is it of good quality? Has it been developed using accepted methods, such as incorporating all available research evidence?
- Will it be credible or acceptable to local policy-makers and practitioners? Are the developers well respected? Did the developers have any conflict of interest?

Having established that a new guideline needs to be developed, you need to go through several preliminary steps. First, you need to determine who should be involved in a development group. There are two categories to consider: the policy-makers and clinicians whose views and behaviour you want the guidelines to influence; and those who will be on the receiving end of the guidelines (for clinical guidelines that will include patients and their carers; for organizational guidelines it will include health care staff). The size of the development group will depend on the method you adopt. Generally, groups are of 10–20 members in size. Additional people can be consulted during the process. Having decided, say, that you want three community health workers to be involved, you have to identify and select specific individuals. They can be randomly or carefully chosen – research suggests that the important factor is a person's 'tribe' (such as community health worker), rather than the particular person chosen.

Second, having assembled your group, each member needs to declare their beliefs about the topic (e.g. 'I think the treatment is excellent and should always be used'). Everyone will have existing views and beliefs. That does not preclude them from participating but it is important for everyone to make known their views to other participants. They should also declare any potential conflict of interest (e.g. a surgeon who earns money doing a certain procedure which is the subject of the guideline). There is no problem in members having strong beliefs or interests as long as the group and, later on, the users of the guideline are aware of it.

Third, the group needs to decide which particular aspects of the guideline topic they are going to focus on. Generally, there are many aspects that could be considered, but too many to be covered realistically. So the group must select those areas where they believe guidelines could have the maximum effect on improving the quality of health care. For example, it might be the way patients are investigated and diagnosed rather than on how best to treat them or how best to help them rehabilitate afterwards.

The process of defining precisely the scope of the guidelines may need to take into account the extent of existing good quality research evidence. So the process has to be iterative. After a preliminary prioritization, it will be necessary to see what research evidence exists. The final decision on scope will be arrived at by considering the groups' priorities in the light of the availability of research evidence.

Reviewing the research evidence

The first thing to do is to check whether anyone else has already reviewed the literature. To be acceptable, a review needs to have been systematic by adopting clear methods for:

- searching the literature
- selecting potential papers
- judging the methodological quality of the studies
- synthesizing the evidence from all the papers selected.

Although *systematic reviews* were developed primarily to consider quantitative research evidence on the effectiveness of health care interventions, they have been developed to encompass economic evaluations and evidence from qualitative studies.

As with guidelines, the number of systematic reviews available is rapidly growing. The pre-eminent organization that undertakes systematic reviews and ensures their rigour is the Cochrane Collaboration. All the reviews its members have published or are currently conducting can be found in its online library (http://www.cochranelibrary.com/cochrane-database-of-systematic-reviews/index.html).

Systematic reviews are widely recognized as reliable sources of information about the effects of health and social care interventions. But as with individual research studies, they can have flaws and can be difficult to interpret. To assist, the Centre for Reviews & Dissemination in the UK has, since 1994, produced and maintained a database providing access to over 13,000 abstracts of quality assessed and critically appraised systematic reviews (http://www.crd.york.ac.uk/CRDWeb/). For inclusion, reviews must meet at least three criteria, of which criteria 1 and 2 below are mandatory:

1 *Were inclusion/exclusion criteria reported that addressed the review question?* A good review should focus on a well-defined question, which

defines the inclusion/exclusion criteria by which decisions are made on whether to include or exclude primary studies. The criteria should relate to the four components of study design, participants, intervention or organization, and outcomes of interest.

2 *Was the search adequate?* This is usually the case if details of electronic database searches and other identification strategies are given. Ideally, details of the search terms used, date, and language restrictions should be presented. In addition, descriptions of hand-searching, attempts to identify unpublished material, and any contact with authors, industry, and research institutes should be provided. The appropriateness of the database(s) searched by the authors should also be considered; for example, if MEDLINE is searched for a review evaluating health promotion, then it is unlikely that all relevant studies will have been located.

3 *Was the validity of the included studies assessed?* Authors should have taken account of study design and quality, either by restricting inclusion criteria, or systematic assessment of study quality. A systematic assessment of the quality of primary studies should include information about the criteria used (e.g. method of randomization, whether outcome assessment was blinded). Authors often use a published checklist or scale, or one that they have designed specifically for their review.

4 *Are sufficient details about the individual included studies presented?* The review should demonstrate that the studies included are suitable to answer the question posed and that a judgement on the appropriateness of the authors' conclusions can be made.

These criteria also serve as advice as to how you should go about creating your own systematic review if no existing ones are suitable. For more detail as to how to conduct a review, you should consult one of the many instruction manuals available. You will find a free one at: http://www.york.ac.uk/media/crd/Systematic_Reviews.pdf.

Combining research evidence with experience

Occasionally in health care there is clear research evidence to indicate the best way of managing a patient or organizing a service. Generally, however, the research evidence is either lacking or of poor quality. Even when the research evidence is of reasonable quality, there is a need to translate it into guidelines for a particular place. That is because the local context must be considered. The latter includes the level of resources, the skill of staff, and the beliefs and attitudes of the local population. You have already seen in Chapter 7 the impact such factors can have. In the Netherlands, Ferket and colleagues (2012) compared guidelines for screening for abdominal aortic aneurysm that had been created in Canada, the USA, and the UK. All three development groups reviewed the same literature but three sets of recommendations differed significantly in several respects, including who should be screened:

- UK: men aged 65–74 years
- Canada: men aged 65–74 years and women over 64 years with multiple risk factors
- USA: men aged 60–85 years and those aged 50–64 with a family history of the condition plus women aged 50–85 years with one risk factor.

The differences partly reflect differences in expenditure on health care between the three countries and the extent of professional autonomy (as you saw in Chapters 1 and 5). This influenced the way the opinions and experience of the members of the guideline development group were combined with the research evidence. Traditionally, groups have been composed of self-appointed 'experts' forming a committee and making decisions in an informal way (without any explicit rules).

✎ **Activity 11.4**

Think about any committees you have been on. What do you think are the dangers of an informal process for decision-making?

Feedback

There are several dangers in relying on an informal process: the most powerful members of the group often dominate and the less confident or less powerful feel (or even fear) they cannot challenge; the reasons for decisions may not be clear; and the group is more likely to arrive at inconsistent decisions.

These concerns have led to the use of formal *consensus development methods*. Of the several methods available, the most commonly used one for developing guidelines is the nominal group technique. It has several forms but the key, common features are that the group members express their views in private using structured questionnaires to indicate their level of agreement with a series of statements about good practice (Raine et al., 2005). The anonymity ensures they do not feel under any pressure from other members. The group then meets to discuss the more controversial issues and to learn the reasons for any points of disagreement. While the aim is to improve the level of agreement within the group, there should be no attempt or pressure for members to agree just for the sake of it. The group is only 'nominal' in the sense that it does not seek to arrive at an explicit group decision (such as through a transparent vote) but allows each member to express their views privately and then forms the group view by combining the individual views.

Summary

You have learnt about the need for explicit, evidence-based guidelines to assure the public they are receiving care of the highest quality, and how reviews of research evidence need to be conducted in a systematic way and then combined with expert wisdom and experience to create guidelines that are appropriate for a specific health care system at a particular time. In the following chapter, you will learn about how guidelines can underpin the assessment of the quality of care.

References

Davies, H. (1999) Falling public trust in health services: implications for accountability, *Journal of Health Services Research and Policy*, 4 (4): 193–4.

Ferket, B.S., Grootenboer, N., Colkesen, E.B., Visser, J.J., van Sambeek, M.R., Spronk, S. et al. (2012) Systematic review of guidelines on abdominal aortic aneurysm screening, *Journal of Vascular Surgery*, 55 (5): 1296–304.

Raine, R., Black, N. and Sanderson, C. (2005) Developing clinical guidelines: a challenge to current methods, *British Medical Journal*, 331 (7517): 631–3.

Sackett, D.L., Rosenberg, W.M., Gray, J.A., Haynes, R.B. and Richardson, W.S. (1996) Evidence based medicine: what it is and what it isn't, *British Medical Journal*, 312 (7023): 71–2.

12 Quality assessment

Overview

In the previous chapter, you learned about how criteria for good quality can be derived from reviewing the research literature and combining that with the views of clinicians and lay people. In this chapter, you will learn about how the quality of services can be assessed. You will consider the range of methods needed, the two principal challenges to assessing effectiveness, the difficulty of assessing whole systems or whole health care organizations, and the need therefore to focus on specific clinical areas and the importance of engaging with clinicians. In Chapter 13, you will complete the journey by considering what action can be taken to improve quality.

Learning objectives

After working through this chapter, you will be able to:

- understand the need for a range of methods when assessing quality
- describe the two key challenges in assessing effectiveness: data quality and case-mix differences
- understand the difficulties of making meaningful comparisons of whole health care systems and health care provider organizations
- explain ways in which the effectiveness of specific services can be rigorously assessed
- understand the need for clinician engagement

Key terms

Case-mix: The mix of cases (patients) that a provider cares for that will inevitably influence the outcome of care (e.g. age, severity, co-morbidity).

Confounder: Characteristics of patients that are associated both with their likelihood of being treated and the likelihood of the outcome (e.g. age, severity).

Critical incident inquiry: A set of procedures used for collecting direct observations of actions that have critical significance and meet methodically defined criteria.

Hospital-wide standardized mortality ratio: The number of deaths in a hospital compared with the number that would be expected (based on the average performance of all hospitals).

Retrospective case record review: Patients' medical records are reviewed to determine if there were any acts of commission (e.g. giving the wrong drug) or of omission (e.g. failing to carry out a test) that caused harm.

Risk (case-mix) adjustment: A statistical process to make allowance for any difference in case-mix between providers when comparing their performance.

History

Performance assessment is not new. In 1750, the board of the British Lying-In Hospital questioned mothers about their stays and took action accordingly: 'Patients' disappointment over rancid caudle [beer and bread], bedbugs, and neglect by the female staff led to immediate investigations and remedies, including firing negligent staff found to be guilty or, on the other hand, prohibiting the complainant from receiving future charity if her charges were discovered to be exaggerated or false.' In the nineteenth century, Florence Nightingale (who was an accomplished statistician as well as a leading reformer of nursing and hospital organization) used quantitative measures to compare the outcomes of London hospitals and this was continued by two surgeons in the early twentieth century: E.W. Groves in Bristol, England, and E.A. Codman in Boston, USA. You have seen in Chapter 1 how, by the 1980s, Arnold Relman considered that a new era of assessment and accountability had arrived centre-stage.

✎ Activity 12.1

Remind yourself of the reasons Relman (1988) gave for the current focus on assessment and accountability.

Feedback

He cited several factors, including:

- the need for cost containment
- advances in health care technology producing new opportunities and ways of delivering care
- evidence of wide variations in the use of health care between geographical populations.

Since then, there has also been a growing awareness of the incidence of iatrogenesis (harm caused by health care). In addition, the rapid development of the internet has meant that members of the public have gained access to lots of medical information resulting in much better informed and, in some cases more critical, patients and their carers.

Range of methods needed

The different domains of quality require different assessment methods, some quantitative and some qualitative. Each has its advantages and limitations. Generally speaking, quantitative methods will provide information on the frequency of events whereas qualitative methods will help understand how and why events occurred.

This can be seen in the assessment of safety, which involves two quantitative and one qualitative approach. Safety can be quantified by getting staff to *prospectively report* any adverse incidents (such as a patient given the wrong drug dose) when they occur, although this depends on staff remembering to report and requires an open, trusting organization in which staff are not punished for admitting to mistakes. In addition, staff can be required to report the occurrence of any harm such as a wound infection or a fracture resulting from a patient falling. The frequency of unsafe care can also be measured using a *retrospective case record review* in which patients' written records are reviewed to determine how often any adverse events or incidents occurred. This should include both acts of commission, such as administering the wrong drug, and acts of omission when there is a failure to deliver care, such as not carrying out an investigation or not giving a patient sufficient fluids.

In contrast, a qualitative approach such as *critical incident inquiries* can be used to study single adverse incidents in depth to understand how they came about (and use the lessons learnt to improve care in future). Such inquiries involve a set of procedures for collecting direct observations of people's behaviour that have critical significance and meet methodically defined criteria.

🖉 Activity 12.2

Assessment of humanity also makes use of quantitative and qualitative approaches. Can you suggest what methods might be used?

Feedback

1 The most commonly used quantitative method is a patient experience survey in which people who have used health services are invited to complete a questionnaire about their experience. This may

include the dignity and respect they were shown, level of privacy, whether they received all the information desired, the quality and choice of food provided (if they were in-patients), how clean the facilities were, and how long they had to wait.

2   Qualitative methods include observation of the way patients are treated, interviews with patients, and focus groups (interviews and discussions with a group of patients).

As you learnt in Chapter 11, it is important to recognize that humanity of care can either seek the patient's experience or their satisfaction with care. The difference is that the latter will be affected by their expectations. So someone might receive poor care but because their expectations are low, they report they are satisfied. Patient experience measures are generally preferred, as they seek to avoid the influence of differences in people's expectations (e.g. older people tend to have lower expectations than younger ones).

Equity of care can only be assessed using quantitative methods. Usually it will use routinely collected data such as hospital administrative data or primary care utilization data. However, such data allow only a crude assessment of the equity of use of services (limited because such data rarely include information on patients' severity). And administrative data do not include much information on outcome (often just whether the patient left hospital dead or alive), so they cannot be used to assess the equity of outcomes.

Even more challenging is assessing the effectiveness of care. It may be possible to use a process measure (such measures are defined in the clinical guidelines you learnt about in Chapter 11) if there is good evidence of an association with a health outcome. For example, it is well established that people who have an acute myocardial infarction (heart attack) benefit from having an angioplasty within 90 minutes. So the proportion of patients receiving angioplasty in that timeframe can be used as a measure of the effectiveness of the services provided. If there is no strong evidence of an association between process (treatment) and outcome, effectiveness can only be assessed by measuring patients' outcomes. In the next section, you will learn about the two principal challenges when assessing effectiveness.

Challenges when assessing effectiveness

Data quality

A key element of any quantitative assessment, regardless of the level of analysis or the use of process or outcome measures is data quality. Four main aspects of data quality (consistency of definitions, completeness, validity, reliability) need to be considered. First is the *lack of consistency of data definitions*.

 ✎   **Activity 12.3**

What difficulties do you think you might encounter in defining the following?

1 a breast-fed infant
2 diabetes
3 length of hospital stay
4 a hospital bed

Feedback

---

1 You would need to define whether you meant exclusively breast-fed or not; and would once a day for a few minutes count as 'breast-fed'?
2 While some conditions are either present or not (e.g. a broken bone), most occur in a wide spectrum of severity from mild and insignificant to severe and life-threatening. When mild, one doctor may diagnose diabetes whereas another may consider the person is still within normal physiological bounds.
3 Length of stay can be defined as starting on arrival at a hospital or arrival on a ward; some hospitals may count a day-case staying eight hours as 'one day' whereas others may not include day-cases as 'admissions'.
4 Beds on wards are straightforward but should beds in emergency rooms be included and when does a trolley become a bed?

Second is the problem of *collecting complete data*. It is almost inevitable that some data will be missing. If this occurs randomly and only occasionally, then it is unlikely to matter. But in some health care systems, missing data is so common as to render the data unfit for assessing performance.

Third, data must be *valid* – that is, provide a true indication of reality. There is some evidence that data may be deliberately distorted to ensure the performance of a service or system appears better than it really is. Such 'gaming' will undermine the validity of assessment.

And fourth, data must be *reliable* – that is, if collected again by the same person (intra-rater reliability) or by someone else (inter-rater reliability), the result would be the same.

Case-mix differences

As you will be aware, the types of patient that different doctors and different institutions care for vary. Sometimes this is deliberate. For example, tertiary care facilities are expected to manage particularly complex and difficult cases. If practitioners' or institutions' performance were to be compared without taking such differences into account, the comparisons would at best be meaningless and at worst misleading. The performance measure (be it process or outcome) needs to take the different mix of cases each provider manages (case-mix) into account by statistical adjustment. This is also referred to as 'risk adjustment' (as you are adjusting for each patient's risk of a good or bad outcome).

Comparisons must, therefore, take into account all the patient characteristics that are known to be associated with the effectiveness of care (e.g. age, severity, comorbidity). These are known as confounding factors and must be adjusted for by means of statistical techniques. Clearly, it is only possible to adjust for the factors that are known to be confounders (there may well be others that we are unaware of such as genetic characteristics) and for which data are available.

✎ Activity 12.4

If there are shortcomings either in data quality or case-mix adjustment, it is likely that the resulting assessments will be challenged, particularly by those with unfavourable assessments. One of the earliest attempts to adopt this approach was cardiac surgery in New York State. As you read the following edited article, written in the 1990s but still pertinent today, make notes on what three criticisms were made and how the author, Ed Hannan, responded.

Measuring hospital outcomes: don't make perfect the enemy of good!

In recent years there has been a proliferation of outcomes research in an attempt to measure the quality of health care. One of the types that has been most popular, and most controversial, is the development and sometimes public dissemination of risk-adjusted adverse outcome rates (usually mortality) for surgical procedures or medical conditions.

... The first public report based on clinical data collected expressly for the purpose of assessing quality was the New York State Cardiac Surgery Report in 1990, which was followed by a similar report on cardiac surgery in Pennsylvania that was released in 1992. These reports, which continue to be produced, present risk-adjusted mortality for surgeons who perform coronary artery bypass grafting (CABG) and for hospitals in which CABG is performed ...

These efforts have been vociferously criticized. Among the reasons given are that the statistical models do not adjust adequately for differences in the pre-operative risks of patients, that the publication of death rates results in perverse incentives regarding treatment decisions that could *have adverse consequences for patients, and that public dissemination results subsequently in over-reporting of risk factors by hospitals that yields an inaccurate risk-adjustment process.*

Inadequacy of risk adjustment

Some of the justification for maintaining that the models are not good enough is that there are large changes in provider risk-adjusted mortality ranks from year to year. Although this is true, the idea that ranks are an important indication of relative quality is merely an ignorant misconception as to how the information is to be used. Hospitals are judged to have different adverse outcome rates only when their risk-adjusted mortalities are found to be statistically different. In fact most, if not all, of the reports I have seen present the outcomes in alphabetical order of provider, rather than in the order of risk-adjusted mortality, so as to discourage improper use of the data in the reports.

Creation of perverse incentives for providers

The only study I am aware of that addresses perverse incentives regarding treatment decisions is a study that concludes that significantly more high-risk New York State patients migrated out of the state to undergo CABG at the Cleveland Clinic during 1989–1993 than during 1980–1988 (Omoigui et al., 1996). However, the time period being used is inaccurate since New York data were released for the first time in December 1990. Also, the average severity of New York State patients at the Cleveland Clinic changed little between 1990 and 1993. Furthermore, the annual number of patients undergoing CABG in New York rose at a fairly steady pace, as did the average pre-operative severity of these patients. A study using Medicare data (which is the only US national database) demonstrated that the proportion of New York patients referred out-of-state for CABG actually declined from 14.8% in 1989 to 11.8% in 1992.

Over-reporting of risk factors

There are undoubtedly perverse incentives associated with reporting the risk factors used to adjust for case mix in a clinical database that is to be used for public dissemination of information, since the sicker a provider's patients appear, the lower the provider's risk-adjusted mortality will be. However, these incentives can be controlled by monitoring data quality. Contrary to allegations that the reported prevalence rates of risk factors in New York have fluctuated wildly, they have actually remained quite stable except for changes related to new definitions for risk factors . . .

Can risk-adjusted outcomes indicate quality of care?

Concerning the use of risk-adjusted outcomes for improving the quality of health care, Brook et al. (1996) state that, with exceptions, the assessment of quality should rely more on process data than outcome data. The main reason given for this opinion is that outcome data may not be sensitive enough since there is not always a poor outcome whenever there is an error in the provision of care. However, these authors also state that there are exceptions to the rule, such as methods of comparing outcomes following CABG. Among the reasons they give for why this is an exception are that there has been extensive research on the best way to adjust statistically for case mix differences, there is strong evidence of the link between quality of care and survival, death is a common enough event to be used as a measure of quality differences, and differences in mortality between providers (hospitals and surgeons) can be assessed relatively soon after surgery.

. . . Also, it is not always known what the optimal processes of care are that lead to better outcomes. The only way to establish this is by observing care with and without what are thought to be optimal processes and demonstrating that the processes lead to better (risk-adjusted) outcomes. After this has been done, it may or may not be advisable to abandon the effort of generating risk-adjusted outcomes.

Conclusions

It is essential that the health services research community continues to improve on hospital and physician quality assessments. There are many areas we need to address, including the theory underlying the statistical models, data quality and accuracy, and preventing or minimizing perverse incentives caused by public release . . . However, there is simply not enough evidence to discontinue these reports, particularly the ones based on clinical data. The best and fastest way to improve them is to search for constructive changes and alternatives while continuing the reports.

Reproduced from Hannan (1998). With permission of the Royal Society of Medicine Press Limited.

Feedback

The three criticisms and Hannan's responses are:

1 Large fluctuations in ranking of hospitals is evidence of inadequate risk adjustment. In response, Hannan points out that ranking is indeed a very unstable indicator and one that should not be used.
2 Creates perverse incentives for providers such as driving high-risk patients out of the system. Hannan shows that the severity of cases treated outside New York State did not change and the proportion that migrated out of state actually fell.
3 Gaming the system by over-reporting patient severity. Hannan states that there is little evidence of this happening and it should be monitored and, if detected, severe sanctions taken.

It is clearly important to consider carefully the quality of data and the adequacy of risk adjustment before making any quantitative comparisons of providers whether looking at effectiveness, safety or the humanity of care. To what extent have meaningful comparisons been carried out either at the macro level of whole health care systems or at the meso level of health care providers (e.g. hospitals)? First, you will learn about the use at the macro level.

Levels of analysis

Macro level

At the end of the twentieth century, some countries and international bodies adopted the ambitious objective of trying to develop single overarching indices that would inform the public about the performance of a whole system. The idea that the complexity and variability of health care could be reduced to a single rating was one that was attractive to politicians. The best known was that carried out by the WHO that appeared in their World Health Report in 2000.

WHO assigned an index measure to each of 191 countries based on four components:

- Population health (using disability adjusted life years and childhood mortality)
- Responsiveness (or the humanity of care including respect, promptness, choice, and access to social support)

Table 12.1 Top ten countries according to the WHO index measure of health system quality

		Overall performance		
Rank	Uncertainty interval	Member state	Index	Uncertainty interval
1	1–5	France	0.994	0.982–1.000
2	1–5	Italy	0.991	0.978–1.000
3	1–6	San Marino	0.988	0.973–1.000
4	2–7	Andorra	0.982	0.966–0.997
5	3–7	Malta	0.978	0.965–0.993
6	2–11	Singapore	0.973	0.947–0.998
7	4–8	Spain	0.972	0.959–0.985
8	4–14	Oman	0.961	0.938–0.985
9	7–12	Austria	0.959	0.946–0.972
10	8–11	Japan	0.957	0.948–0.965

Source: WHO (2000).

- Fairness in financial contributions
- Efficiency

Those countries that appeared at the top of the resulting league table are shown in Table 12.1.

 Activity 12.5

What concerns would you have about the validity of comparisons of the quality of a health care system based on this approach?

Feedback

1   All the components were dependent on national data, which, even in high-income countries, is often incomplete and inaccurate. The use of three decimal points for the index gives an unwarranted suggestion of accuracy.
2   It is not clear why some components are included in the index (e.g. choice of provider is seen as a positive attribute). This reveals the ideological values of the authors.
3   The health of a population is only partly a reflection of the performance of its health services – it is more to do with socio-economic, nutritional, and environmental factors.
4   As you have learnt in Chapter 10, efficiency should not be considered as a dimension of quality.
5   A country's ranking in the world league table will depend crucially on the relative importance ascribed to each component. For example, if population health was considered the most important outcome, you would arrive at a different rank order than if you considered responsiveness as more important.

At the time, proponents argued that despite its shortcomings the index scores and league table of countries helped encourage discussion of health care systems. It is not known if that occurred and whether any benefit resulted, but it is telling that WHO have not repeated the exercise.

Attempts to generate overall ratings for a complex entity like a health care system assume that disparate factors such as the cleanliness of a hospital, the waiting time in the emergency room, and post-operative mortality can sensibly be bolted together to create a composite index. Such a concern has led to other attempts that focus on one particular aspect of health care. In 2015, *The Economist* magazine published an international comparison of the provision of end-of-life care based on five components: palliative and health care environment, human resources, community engagement, affordability, and quality. Again, the results will depend crucially on the relative weighting on each component, which is inherently a political or value judgement, not one that can be based on objective scientific evidence. For example, if affordability is seen as far more important than quality, a country's rating will change.

Meso level

Similar attempts to devise ways of assessing the quality of health care organizations within a country have been pursued over the past two decades. The most commonly used approach has been to assess the quality of a hospital on the basis of its mortality rate adjusted for its case-mix – a hospital-wide standardized mortality ratio (SMR). This compares the number of deaths in a hospital to the number that would be expected (based on average performance). Hospitals are then compared to identify statistical outliers, as the example from the East of England illustrates (Figure 12.1).

Although this metric has become popular in many high-income countries in recent years with some politicians, managers, and the public, it has been criticized by many clinicians and most health services researchers for three main reasons:

1 Although not socially desirable, one of the roles of hospitals is as a place to die (true for 50 per cent of deaths in England), so conceptually it is an inappropriate basis for an indicator of quality.
2 Hospital-wide SMRs partly reflect the proportion of deaths in an area that occur in hospital (which, for example, varies from 40 to 70 per cent in England).
3 SMRs are derived from routine administrative data, the quality of which is inadequate for this use.

In addition, there are serious concerns about the accuracy of the case-mix adjustment that is possible. This was apparent when the State of Massachusetts in the USA commissioned a study from David Shahian and colleagues at Harvard University in 2010, which demonstrated that comparisons of 23 hospitals depended entirely on the way the SMRs were calculated (Shahian et al., 2010). Comparing four different commercially available methods, the SMRs for four hospitals were found to be significantly higher than expected according to one method but lower than expected using a different method. As a result, the state government concluded that the method 'was so flawed that officials do not believe it would be useful to hospitals and patients and could harm public trust in government'. Despite this, other countries have continued to adopt hospital-wide SMRs.

The good news is that other approaches to assessing the quality of health care organizations that are not subject to the same problems are

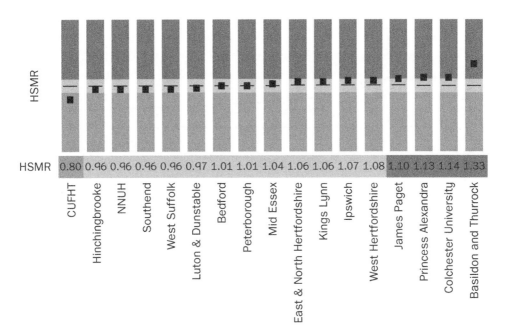

Figure 12.1 Hospital-wide standardized mortality ratios for 17 hospital trusts in the East of England
Source: Flowers (2009).

available. These methods do not try to create an overall measure for an organization. They recognize the complexity and diversity of patients and health care and instead focus on specific patient groups (such as people experiencing a heart attack or diagnosed with diabetes) or clinical areas (such as a cardiology department or a critical care unit). This reduces the differences in case-mix when comparing hospitals and allows more appropriate and specific measures of quality to be used. Another advantage is that in high-income countries, it is increasingly common for clinicians to use and contribute to specialist clinical databases as part of their routine practice (in addition to their patients being included in administrative databases). Clinical databases are usually designed by clinicians, which ensures they are clinically credible and have the trust and engagement of clinicians. They include detailed and accurate data on case-mix, containing all the important known confounding factors, so it is possible to adjust the patients' outcomes adequately for making meaningful comparisons of providers. An example of comparisons of about 200 adult critical care units in the UK can be seen in Figure 12.2. (This is a funnel plot in which a ratio of 1.0 is the mean. Ratios above 1.0 mean there were more deaths than expected; below 1.0 means fewer than expected. The dotted curves are two standard deviations from the mean; the solid curves are three standard deviations.) As can be seen, three units have SMRs that are more than three standard deviations above the expected (something that

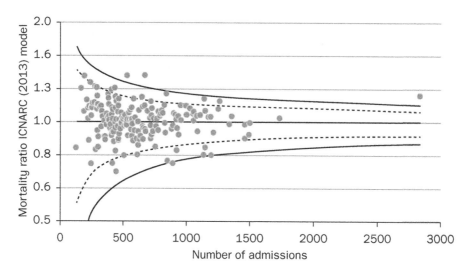

Figure 12.2 Funnel plot of standardized mortality ratios for adult critical care units in the UK in 2013
Source: Intensive Care National Audit and Research Centre (2015).

would only be expected by chance in one in 1000 units), thus warranting close scrutiny by clinicians and managers.

Quality assessment in low- and middle-income countries

Most of the discussion of examples of quality assessment in this chapter has been oriented to high-income countries in which there is widespread availability of computer-based data collection. But it would be wrong to conclude that assessment of the quality of health services in low- and middle-income countries is not possible. The following is an extract from an article by Lynne Franco and colleagues (2002) based on their experience of assessing quality (referred to as performance) in Malawi. They comment on the strengths and weaknesses of four common assessment methods.

Methods for assessing quality of provider performance in developing countries

Observation of provider performance using a checklist

Observation is generally considered as a gold standard for other assessment methods, although there appear to be few empirical studies to validate this. Information derived from observation, when recorded on a structured checklist simultaneously with the provider's actions by an independent observer, provides one of the most complete and reliable pictures of what providers do. This method does not rely on the provider's or the client's memory. However, observers may be unable to discern performance of mental tasks, such as using information collected during history and physical examination of the patient to reach a diagnosis. In addition, observed performance may not represent routine performance if providers modify their behaviour while being observed, and providers may not perform in a consistent manner with every patient they encounter.

Exit interviews with patients or caretakers about provider performance

The reliability of exit interview data depends on the memory of the patient or lay carer, how much attention was paid to the provider's actions, knowledge, and expectations about what the provider should be doing, and comfort with talking to an interviewer. However, if conducted without provider knowledge, exit interviews may capture routine performance. Such interviews could provide a clinically trained interviewer with the opportunity to re-examine the patient to assess accuracy of the diagnosis, although such an examination would add time and other costs to this method, and have some of its own methodological problems.

Reviewing patient or health facility records to assess provider performance

Record reviews, commonly used in industrialized countries, allow retrospective assessment of routine provider performance. Limited only by availability and quality of data, record review can assess a large number of cases, and enables review of severely ill cases or rarer conditions. Yet in developing countries, medical records rarely record findings used to make a diagnosis or any instructions given to the patient. In many outpatient settings, if any records are maintained, they either go home with the patient (e.g. immunization cards or Under-Five cards, etc.) or are health centre patient registers that record only the patient's age, sex, domicile, diagnosis, and treatment given.

Interviews with providers about their performance

Provider interviews or self-reports supply information about what providers know, not necessarily what they routinely do. They can, however, furnish information about how providers interpret information from the history and physical examination of the patient and how they would manage severe cases or referrals.

The formulation of interview questions will also affect the results obtained. Spontaneous responses to open-ended questions (e.g. 'What questions do you ask a patient presenting with cough?') are likely to underestimate what providers do, both for tasks they do not perform often, or for tasks they perform so often that performance becomes unconscious. Probing to stimulate memory or providing fixed choices on self-report can also stimulate responses corresponding to what the provider thinks is the expected answer.

From Franco, L.M., Franco, C., Kumwenda, N. and Nkhoma, W. (2002) Methods for assessing quality of provider performance in developing countries, *International Journal of Quality in Health Care*, 14 (suppl. 1): 17–24, with permission of Oxford University Press.

Engaging clinicians and institutions in quality assessment

The purpose of quality assessment is ultimately to stimulate improvements in the quality of care that the public receives. While many people can contribute to that aim, it will only be successful if those providing care – doctors, nurses, physiotherapists, etc. – together with their managers, are engaged with the way their services are being assessed. Without that, the best-designed approaches to assessment will have little or no influence.

🖉 Activity 12.6

The importance of clinician engagement is described in this edited extract from a paper by one British (James Mountford) and one Canadian (Kaveh Shojania) physician. What reasons do the authors suggest for the reluctance of many clinicians to engage in quality assessment?

Refocusing quality measurement to best support quality improvement: local ownership of quality measurement by clinicians

Legitimate debate should exist around which measures to choose in any given situation, how best to capture patients' journeys across different clinical settings, the technical merits and drawbacks of specific measures, and so on. However, little progress will occur until clinicians and institutions (hospitals, group practices, etc.) take ownership of these issues and play active roles in measuring their performance.

Across countries, most clinicians – especially physicians – and healthcare institutions have regarded performance measurement primarily as an administrative burden. They have seen measurement as a task with marginal relevance to patient care imposed by outside forces – insurers, regulators, government agencies – rather than viewing measurement as an important ingredient in improving patient care. However, the best performing healthcare organisations take local ownership of quality measurement, and they do so proactively, rather than reactively in response to external demands . . .

When taking care of a patient, the routine of clinical assessment, formulating a diagnosis and instituting a management plan is second nature for clinicians, who then periodically check in to make sure that tests and investigations requested have been performed and consult the patient to see if they are improving. Similarly, for a health system, an initial assessment is made to reach a 'diagnosis' using various quality and productivity measures, then changes are initiated to address problems identified and as 'treatment' progresses, these measures are repeated – while also checking in with the 'patient'. Just as the treatments serve no purpose if patients do not experience better health, so is the case with our systems of care.

Research over past decades has repeatedly shown that suboptimal systems of care hold back the delivery of effective care to patients. Thus, clinicians can no longer maintain that poorly organised systems are somebody else's problem. Clinicians who truly care about the outcomes of their patients must turn their attention to the systems of care in which they deliver patient care. Central to improving a system is defining and tracking those measures that best describe that system's performance.

Physicians must engage in quality measurement and improvement efforts proactively and must do so with real ownership. Failure to do so will perpetuate the current problems which directly impact the care of individual patients and will also lead to increasing imposition of a quality measurement agenda by external bodies. In fact, in this regard, clinicians have too often espoused contradictory excuses for not participating in activities related to quality measurement and improvement. On the one hand, they have claimed that they are too busy taking care of patients and that system issues are somebody else's problem. On the other hand, whenever someone else proposes an initiative to measure or improve quality, clinicians criticize it as clinically unsound.

The focus on healthcare quality in the past decade has so far been relatively kind to clinicians. Despite numerous studies documenting how often and how far patient care falls short of best practice, emphasis has mostly been placed on the need to improve the systems in which care is delivered, rather than on the competence or professionalism of clinicians. While systems certainly need improving, clinicians must also do their part in improving systems. Vigorous performance measurement plays a vital role in improving systems, and here clinicians must not drag their feet, grudgingly accepting or passively resisting metrics imposed from outside. Rather they must participate actively in the development of metrics, joining a dialogue with colleagues, patients, payers and regulators of healthcare to articulate how quality is best described for each clinical setting, service or pathway.

If clinicians do not respond to the growing calls to make the measurement of healthcare quality a core part of their professional activities and ethos, the perception of clinicians as victims of poorly designed systems may change to a less charitable one. Clinicians risk being seen as part of the problem and at that point it may be too late for them to lead (or even to participate meaningfully) in the development of performance metrics. They will simply have to play along with externally developed metrics, with all the problems these have entailed in the past. Most importantly, patients will not be well served if clinicians do not embrace the measurement and improvement of quality as a core part of their routine work.

From Mountford, J. and Shojania, K. (2012) Refocusing quality measurement to best support quality improvement: local ownership of quality measurement by clinicians, *BMJ Quality and Safety*, 21 (6): 519–23, with permission from BMJ Publishing Group Ltd.

Feedback

The authors suggest several reasons for the reluctance of many clinicians to engage in quality assessment, including: clinicians viewing quality assessment as an administrative burden, of marginal value to patient care, imposed by outside agencies and simply not having the time to engage.

In the next chapter, you will learn about the different ways that clinicians, managers, policy-makers, and regulators can respond to the findings of quality assessment to stimulate improvements.

Summary

You have seen how crucial it is that health care providers (and to a lesser extent purchasers) maintain public trust in their services. This has been the case for over 200 years. You have learnt about the need for a range of methods, both quantitative and qualitative, and how the former is the principal approach to assessing the effectiveness of care. The limitations of trying to assess whole systems or health care organizations and the need to shift the focus to particular patient groups or interventions were discussed. Finally, the need to engage clinicians in this process if it is to be effective in stimulating quality improvement was highlighted.

References

Brook, R.H., McGlynn, E.A. and Cleary, P.D. (1996) Quality of health care. Part 2: measuring quality of care, New England Journal of Medicine, 335 (13): 966–70.

Economist Intelligence Unit (2015) The 2015 Quality of Death Index: Ranking palliative care across the world. London: The Economist. Available at: http://www.eiuperspectives.economist.com/sites/default/files/2015%20EIU%20Quality%20of%20Death%20Index%20Oct%202029%20FINAL.pdf (accessed 19 April 2016).

Flowers, J. (2009) Hospital Mortality and the Epidemiology of In Hospital Death. Available at: http://www.thehealthwell.info/node/99164 (accessed 6 April 2016).

Franco, L.M., Franco, C., Kumwenda, N. and Nkhoma, W. (2002) Methods for assessing quality of provider performance in developing countries, International Journal of Quality in Health Care, 14 (suppl. 1): 17–24.

Hannan, E.L. (1998) Measuring hospital outcomes: don't make perfect the enemy of good!, Journal of Health Services Research and Policy, 3 (2): 67–9.

Intensive Care National Audit and Research Centre (ICNARC) (2015) Annual Quality Report 2013/14 for Adult, General Critical Care. Available at: https://onlinereports.icnarc.org/Reports/2015/1/annual-quality-report-201314-for-adult-general-icu-icuhdu-critical-care (accessed 19 April 2016).

Mountford, J. and Shojania, K. (2012) Refocusing quality measurement to best support quality improvement: local ownership of quality measurement by clinicians, BMJ Quality and Safety, 21 (6): 519–23.

Omoigui, N.A., Miller, D.P., Brown, K.J., Annan, K., Cosgrove, D., III, Lytle, B. et al. (1996) Outmigration for coronary bypass surgery in an era of public dissemination of clinical outcomes, *Circulation*, 93 (1): 27–33.

Relman, A.S. (1988) Assessment and accountability: the third revolution in medical care, *New England Journal of Medicine*, 319 (18): 1220–2.

Shahian, D.M., Wolf, R.E., Iezzoni, L.I., Kirle, L. and Normand, S.-L.T. (2010) Variability in the measurement of hospital-wide mortality rates, *New England Journal of Medicine*, 363: 2530–9.

World Health Organization (WHO) (2000) *The World Health Report 2000. Health Systems: Improving performance.* Geneva: WHO.

13 Improving quality of care

Overview

In the last three chapters you have learnt about the dimensions of quality, how to define good quality care, and how to assess quality, in particular the strengths and limitations of quantitative measures. In this final chapter you will learn about the wide variety of interventions available and the factors necessary to achieve improvements in quality.

Learning objectives

After working through this chapter, you will be able to:

- describe the range of interventions that have been used
- explain the key roles that patients can play in quality improvement
- explain ways in which staff can be supported and helped to improve services

Key terms

Accreditation: Voluntary schemes run by independent bodies assessing attributes of an organization largely based on structural characteristics rather than processes or outcomes.

Clinical pathway: The route or journey a patient follows from lay referral to treatment.

Co-production: The combination of professionals and patients in their clinical management, particularly for long-term conditions.

Litigation: Legal action taken by patients against health care providers for alleged malpractice.

Redesign (re-engineer): Changes to the way services are organized at a micro-level (e.g. a health centre, ward, clinic).

> **Shared decision-making:** The sharing of decisions between professionals and patients, which can be aided by computer software incorporating probabilities of different outcomes and patients' utilities.
>
> **Total quality management:** An approach to quality improvement that involves the commitment of all members of an organization to meeting the needs of its external and internal customers.

Mapping quality improvement interventions

The methods of quality assessment you learnt about in Chapter 12 are not, by themselves, sufficient to lead to improvements in quality. Feedback of information to practitioners and providers makes them aware of how their services compare with those provided by others. It aims to stimulate clinicians and managers to improve. Often that is not easy because institutional rigidity must be overcome. Most people and most organizations are reluctant to change the way they function. Unless rigid boundaries between different clinical professions (such as between psychiatrists and psychologists, doctors and nurses) and established attitudes to how patients should be managed (such as not recognizing the contribution that patients can make to their own treatment) can be overcome, change is impossible. Indeed, 'un-freezing' the status quo is probably the hardest part of bringing about change. The principal contribution of quality assessment is to help this process by holding up a mirror to staff and institutions to enable them to see the need for change.

Once the need for change is accepted, a wide variety of interventions are available to help shape the future. In many countries, quality improvement (also referred to as service or performance improvement) methods have been introduced gradually, each new one being added to existing activities (Batalden and Davidoff, 2007). The result in most countries has been a jungle of uncoordinated activities that can cause confusion, consume excessive resources, and antagonize the very people (clinicians) whose behaviour you want to change.

Before you learn about the interventions available, you need to consider the way in which health care providers apply them. Traditionally, providers would select a method and carry out a one-off activity. For example, they might decide to review the quality of the food being provided for in-patients or the rate of obstetric mishaps. This would be followed up with an intervention, such as a retraining session or the issuance of guidelines. This traditional approach can be effective but it tends to result in small isolated patches of improvement. To achieve large-scale transformation, the underlying issues in an organization or system must be addressed in an on-going approach in which the culture is committed to quality improvement. Change and achieving high quality have to become an integral part of the organization with all staff committed to the purpose. This is known as *total quality management* (or continuous quality improvement) and it recognizes that the culture of the organization is crucial to achieving high quality.

Total quality management is based on the conviction that high quality services are those that best meet the needs of most customers. While the obvious 'customers' are the patients being served, there are also internal customers. The latter are staff who depend on the services of other staff (e.g. ward nurses depend on porters to move patients; doctors depend on staff in diagnostic departments to carry out tests). In this approach, quality is the responsibility of all staff, not just those employed to undertake quality improvement. It presupposes that there are clear and proper long-term organizational goals which all staff are aware of and committed to. The organization needs to establish good communication throughout so that staff are kept informed of their own performance and achievements. The emphasis is on learning from experiences, supporting those who need assistance, and avoiding a blame culture in which staff feel the need to hide any faults through fear of punishment.

✎ Activity 13.1

Turning to the improvement interventions that exist, spend a few minutes writing down all the approaches to improving quality that you are aware of in your own country.

Feedback

You may have included some of the following, which are commonly used around the world: regulation of clinicians; accreditation of facilities; litigation for malpractice; financial incentives; inspections; inquiries; education; redesign of service delivery.

The wide range of interventions available can be categorized into five main approaches, each of which you will consider in the rest of this chapter:

• education
• incentives
• redesign
• regulation
• legal action.

Education

Education (or re-education) tends to be the first response of clinicians and managers following the identification of poor quality care. However, in general, staff know what they should be doing. Problems arise when they act differently, such as taking short-cuts to speed up their work. Providing educational inputs to staff in such situations will not have any impact and might actually alienate the very people you are trying to engage.

Having said that, in some situations it will be appropriate to establish (or re-establish) what everyone should be doing. There are many ways of educating people but the traditional approaches to teaching, such as lectures and seminars, while fine for imparting knowledge, have little to contribute when the aim is to change people's behaviour. Instead, the most frequently used approaches in quality improvement are the issuance of guidelines and, in countries with computing facilities, computer-based reminders.

You learnt about the development of guidelines in Chapter 11. Guidelines are often fairly extensive documents, so it is necessary to create short practical versions that people will have time to use. It is now standard practice to publish guidelines in three forms: an extensive account providing all the background information and the evidence on which they are based; a shorter version for the relevant health care workers; and an even shorter version for patients that avoids jargon and non-essential technical detail.

In countries with widespread computing facilities in their health care systems, it is possible to build in automatic reminders so that good quality care does not depend on a health care worker having to remember key events. For example, many child health services have a database of all the children they are responsible for, such that when a child is due for an immunization or developmental check, the computer lets everyone know. This can help ensure high coverage and reduce the risk of delayed detection of treatable problems. Another example is automatic alerts if a doctor prescribes a drug that might interact adversely with another drug the patient is on or to which the patient is known to be allergic.

Education should not be confined to staff. The benefit to patients with long-term conditions of playing an active role in managing their condition is now widely accepted. As you read in Chapter 8, there is an increasing focus on educating and supporting patients as the 'co-producers' of their own health. In many countries, self-management programmes have been instituted to help patients develop understanding and expertise in how to manage their condition. This can improve patients' self-esteem, ensure the multiple services such patients receive are better integrated, improve outcomes, and reduce costs. Everybody benefits.

Greater involvement and partnership with patients can also result in benefits for patients with acute conditions through the use of shared decision-making. Although much can be achieved without computing, software applications can provide sophisticated methods for individualized risk prediction based on a combination of the best scientific evidence of effectiveness and patients' own utilities (values) regarding the different outcomes that might result from treatment. For example, a woman with menstrual bleeding problems can be assisted in making the best decision for herself by using software that asks her about the value she puts on such outcomes as a reduction in symptoms, maintaining her fertility, and having some urinary incontinence. In a review in 2010, Elwyn and colleagues identified 55 randomized trials on the impact of shared decision-making, mostly for surgical operation for non-life-threatening conditions. The studies showed that patients were better informed and less passive, had better adherence to their chosen treatment, and were 25 per cent less likely to opt for surgery (though this might only result in delaying the decision rather than never having an operation).

Activity 13.2

The impact of shared decision-making for several types of surgical operations was reported in a systematic review by O'Connor and colleagues (2009). Figure 13.1 shows the results for nine studies from the USA and two from the UK[1]. The decision to opt for surgery among those receiving standard care is compared with those taking part in shared decision-making using decision aids. Summarize their main findings.

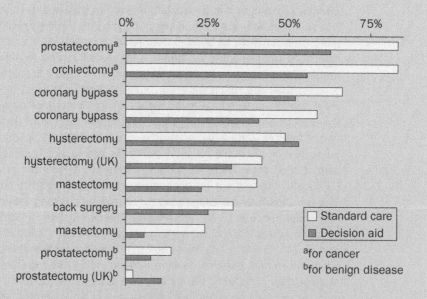

Figure 13.1 Impact of use of decision aids on demand for certain surgical operations in nine US studies and two UK studies

Source: Based on O'Connor et al. (2009).

---

[1]Full details and references of the included studies can be found in O'Connor et al. (2009).

Feedback

Shared decision-making resulted in fewer patients opting for surgery in the USA for all procedures with the exception of hysterectomy. This even included surgery for cancer of the prostate and testes. In the UK, shared decision-making resulted in fewer hysterectomies but more prostatectomies (for benign disease). The latter might be a consequence of a pre-existing low rate of surgery suggesting that patients valued the operation more highly than their surgeons.

Despite the benefits of shared decision-making, implementation has proved difficult and slow in most countries. It is still rarely used on a routine basis. While this is partly because of the lack of good scientific evidence on many treatment options, it is probably more to do with clinicians' lack of enthusiasm, as its adoption requires a change of clinical culture regarding the relationship between doctors and patients.

Incentives

Incentives come in two main forms: they may either be financial (such as extra pay for carrying out an activity) or socio-behavioural (i.e. appealing to workers' desire to be well regarded by their colleagues and peers). The other key distinction is between incentives that are positive (rewarding good quality) or negative (penalizing poor quality).

In general, professionals respond more to socio-behavioural incentives than financial ones, a fact you should be familiar with given what you have learnt about the nature of professions in Chapter 5 (Biller-Andorno and Lee, 2013). Professionals put great store on what their peers think of them. Most people want to be respected within their own 'tribe'. However, financial incentives can be effective in achieving some discrete change, such as encouraging community health workers to increase immunization rates or the use of impregnated bed nets to prevent malaria (Gopalan et al., 2014). It is also important to recognize that people tend to respond more to positive incentives (e.g. nurse of the week award) than negative incentives, which inculcate fear of the consequences.

Incentives can also be targeted at organizations, such as hospitals, which respond to financial benefits. In all health care systems, providers can only survive if they attract business for which they are reimbursed. In essence, this is a financial incentive. Purchasers can use this as an inducement to improve the quality of care. For example, the level of payment can depend on how well patients are managed using measures such as adherence to clinical guidelines about the appropriate use of investigations and the choice of which drugs are prescribed (e.g. use of cheap generic drugs rather than more expensive proprietary products). Increasingly, attempts are being made to base payments on outcomes as part of the quest to develop 'value-based health care', although this is limited by the lack of outcome measurements for many activities. As you saw in Chapter 12, this is changing in some countries as sophisticated clinical databases are being introduced (such as Quality Registers in Sweden and National Clinical Audits in England).

As with educational interventions, it is important not to forget the potential for driving quality improvement through the involvement of patients. Finance can motivate people to take up preventive measures such as screening. Some countries have considered making social security payments dependent on the use of health care, such as antenatal care for pregnant women and rehabilitation services for illicit drug users. This can be successful but is the subject of political debate regarding individuals' rights and the state being coercive through adopting compulsory treatment policies. While rules and compulsion are often used in public health (such as age restrictions on smoking or drinking alcohol), they are rarely if ever used in personal health care.

✎ Activity 13.3

One common means of trying to improve patients' appropriate use of health care is the imposition of co-payments (charges, deductibles). What might be the benefits and the risks of such an approach?

Feedback

As discussed in Chapter 7, co-payments will deter patients from 'misusing' services and thus reduce inappropriate demand on health services such as emergency rooms. It will also contribute to funds for health care.

The risk is that co-payments are just as likely to put off people from seeking appropriate care as inappropriate care. This could result in patients' health worsening and health care systems experiencing more severely ill patients when they do eventually seek help.

Redesign

One of the most common reasons poor quality care occurs is the way clinical services are organized within a provider (health centre, community nursing service, hospital). A frequent problem is the lack of a clear clinical pathway (the route that a patient follows from their initial demand for care). Common problems include duplication of services, unacceptable delays, patients being managed in the wrong part of the system, and poor communication between different practitioners and providers. While such problems may be manifest in numerous ways, there are four broad ways of reorganizing:

- Change the availability of a service (e.g. introduce a list of essential drugs or a hospital limiting the drugs available to avoid doctors using expensive ones when cheaper alternatives exist).
- Change access to a service (e.g. permit primary care doctors to request tests directly rather than having to refer the patient to a specialist first; introduce telemedicine or telehealth so that patients and professionals can monitor progress without the patient having to attend a clinic).
- Change staff responsibilities (e.g. nurses taking over blood pressure checks from doctors).
- Pre-authorization and concurrent review (e.g. a surgeon has to get permission from the purchaser of the service, such as an insurance fund, before operating; requests for diagnostic tests must specify the clinical justification and be approved by a diagnostic specialist).

The scope for redesigning (or re-engineering as it is sometimes called) the processes of health care is enormous (Hoffman and Emanuel, 2013). You have already learnt about one option, that of staff substitution, in Chapter 5. One of the attractions of these approaches is that not only are the staff often already well aware of the shortcomings of their service, but they also have ideas as to how it could be improved. For example, if there are long delays for patients waiting in a clinic, the receptionist is likely to be able to identify a solution. Another example is the overuse of diagnostic investigations by trainee doctors because of worries that their seniors will criticize them if the results are not available. Involving staff in redesigning services will result in their commitment and ownership of the solution. Managers should avoid the temptation to pay external consultants (often large amounts of money) to tell them what changes to make. Instead, they should invest their limited, precious resources in enhancing the skills of their own staff in analysing and improving services. This is akin to the proverb: 'give a man a fish and you feed him for a day; teach a man to fish and you feed him for a lifetime'. In addition, by involving staff, their commitment and ownership are obtained and any changes are more likely to be welcomed and accepted.

There are several formal methods underpinning service redesign. Although they differ from one another in key respects, they share a common theme of systematic analysis of the situation followed by the adoption of a structured approach to change. One of the best known is the *Plan, Do, Study, Act* cycle in which each of the four stages is followed in sequence and then repeated as many times as is necessary to achieve change: Plan – the change to be tested or implemented; Do – carry out the change; Study – data before and after the change and reflect on what was learned; and Act – plan the next change cycle or full implementation.

Some approaches have been adopted from manufacturing industries that seek to achieve perfection with no defective products (e.g. *Six sigma* used by Motorola and General Electric in which their factories seek to reduce the probability of errors to fewer than six standard deviations below the average). Given the differences between manufacturing and service industries, it is unclear how realistic the goal is as it seeks to reduce adverse events to less than 3.4 per million. However, its value is probably as an aspiration to encourage improvement. Another approach adopted from manufacturing is known as *Lean* (developed by Toyota) in that it seeks to avoid any unnecessary activities that could impair the efficiency of the production process. By analysing each step in the clinical management of patients, it maps their pathway and identifies such unwanted features as delays, inappropriate care or waste. It focuses on reducing what patients would define as 'defects' in the system.

Finally, there is a more quantitative approach known as *statistical process control*, in which data on a health care process (such as use of a diagnostic test or length of hospital stay) or an outcome (such as wound infections) is continuously monitored to detect any variation from expectations. It seeks to spot, as quickly as possible, any unjustified (special cause) variation, distinguishing it from the inevitable natural (common cause) variation. Action to understand the reason and correct any problem can then be initiated before further poor quality care occurs.

All of these approaches are thought to have a greater impact if the organization is part of a 'collaborative' – that is, a group of providers addressing the same problem together and learning from each other. The emphasis is on learning rather than on competition as to which provider can be the best.

Regulation

All health care systems use some form of regulation aimed at individual practitioners, institutions or both. In most countries, the basic education of each profession is controlled by a professional regulatory body to ensure all training establishments and courses meet minimum requirements. As you know from Chapter 5, this fulfils one of the characteristics of a profession, that of self-regulation. After basic training, most countries *license* new doctors, nurses or other professions, so as to control who can practise. Licensing is clearly essential to reassure the public. In addition, those who choose to specialize will, in many countries, be required to be *certified* that they are fit for specialist practice. Once licensed, how long clinicians are allowed to practise for varies between countries. Traditionally, professionals were granted the right to practise for life but increasingly high-income countries are imposing some form of regular *revalidation*. The aim is to ensure professionals remain up to date and to assure both employers and the public that they are still fit to practise. As yet there is no evidence as to how effective this is in improving the quality of care (Cayton and Webb, 2014).

Regulation of institutions has grown considerably and now can occupy a lot of managers' time. The most basic form is *accreditation*, which can apply not only to providing services but also aspects such as training programmes (e.g. determining whether or not a provider is a suitable place for training nurses). Accreditation tends to focus on the structural aspects (such as staffing levels and equipment) rather than on processes or outcomes. Seeking accreditation is usually voluntary and requires the institution to pay to have its application processed.

✎ Activity 13.4

There is a lack of rigorous evidence that accreditation improves quality. From what you learnt in Chapter 12, why might that be so?

Feedback

Accreditation concentrates on structural characteristics that may have no strong association with processes (e.g. shorter waiting times, better communication) or outcomes (e.g. lower mortality, better quality of life).

A less common approach is for governments to regulate the provision and location of expensive technology or highly specialist services through *certification*. This aims to ensure greater geographical equity, avoid wasteful duplication of services, and avoid the creation of low-volume providers who may not gain enough experience to produce good outcomes.

One of the most frequently used approaches is *inspection*. Over the past 200 years this has become more sophisticated. Today, inspectorates will make use of complex data, staff surveys, patients' views as well as interviewing managers, staff and patients during their visit. Inspections may be regular or routine so all institutions can expect to be subjected to such scrutiny. Alternatively, inspections may be carried out selectively when concerns have been raised with the regulator. In either case, visits might be announced or unannounced. The danger of the former is that providers take special measures to present an unrepresentative image (e.g. ensure more staff than normal are working). As with accreditation, there is no rigorous evidence that inspections have a lasting impact on improving quality.

The final method of regulation is the use of *targets*, such as imposing maximum waiting times for patients to be seen or admitted. These appear to have been successful, particularly if the consequence of failing to meet the target leads to loss of income or reputation. In some systems, even managers' jobs can be put at risk. One consequence is that targets encourage providers to focus all their attention on that topic which may be at the expense of other aspects of their services, which, may, as a result, deteriorate.

In addition, staff may alter their behaviour to meet a target but in a way that brings no benefit to patients or might even harm patients. An example of such 'gaming' is to admit patients to hospital from an emergency room unnecessarily just to ensure no one waits longer than a target time period. This is an example of a 'perverse incentive', a good intention that actually proves to be counter-productive and reduces the quality of care provided.

As with other approaches to quality improvement, it is difficult to determine the effect of regulation. A review published in 2009 of 54 studies, mostly in the USA, suggested that there was only limited evidence of the effectiveness of regulation confined to targets for reducing waiting times and some inspections motivating short-term change. Some potential adverse aspects also need to be considered (Black, 2015). Regulation can be expensive, it needs to be repeated frequently as judgements become out of date, it can antagonize those regulated and create resistance, and can be discredited by false negatives (i.e. providers judged as doing well that are later found to be providing poor quality care). One additional danger is that those being regulated can gain control over the regulating body. Avoidance of this hazard depends on regulators remaining detached and not being unduly influenced by those they are assessing (who may be colleagues in the same profession or specialty). There is the danger of those being regulated defining the criteria by which they will be assessed. For example, surgeons may decide that they should be assessed solely in terms of their post-operative mortality, whereas patients might also want to see the surgeons' communication skills included.

Regulation should therefore be used sparingly and confined to where it is essential (such as licensing professionals), otherwise it may be counter-productive, creating resistance among the very people whom you hope to change.

Legal action

Of the five broad approaches to quality improvement, the use of legal action probably varies the most internationally. It tends to reflect the legal culture of a country – that is, the propensity to resort to the courts to resolve issues. Laws may relate to the requirements for institutions to ensure that patients and staff are safe and can provide high quality care; for example, laws governing health and safety, minimizing the risk of fire in buildings, and protecting staff employment rights (e.g. working hours and pay). These have either a direct or indirect influence on the quality of care through ensuring staff are satisfied (which is known to be associated with better patient experience and outcomes).

There is a debate as to whether litigation (or the threat of it) helps improve the quality of care or harms it. Some argue that fear leads practitioners and providers to be 'defensive' and avoid taking risks. This may not be in a patient's interest. For example, it is argued that the high rates of caesarean sections in some countries may be because if an obstetrician perceives there to be a risk in leaving a woman to try to deliver vaginally, he or she will prefer to avoid that risk and deliver the baby by caesarean section. While such behaviour is understandable, it may result in poorer quality care (i.e. delivering babies by caesarean section rather than giving mothers the opportunity to deliver normally). It may also divert resources from the many to the few. Another danger is that fear of being subject to legal action may create workforce shortages with, for example, doctors reluctant to enter specialties with a high incidence of litigation and, therefore, high insurance costs.

Does quality improvement work?

The lack of rigorous scientific evidence on the benefits of quality improvement reflects partly that relatively little research has been conducted and partly the methodological difficulties in applying traditional positivist methods of evaluation. It is often not appropriate to experiment with quality improvement interventions, such as using randomized controlled trials. For example, it would be impossible to introduce forms of licensing or certification for only some practitioners. The other obstacle is that only those providers and practitioners who are interested in improving quality will choose to participate in a trial, so participants will be reluctant to be in a control arm in which the intervention is not available. Thus, the very act of random allocation of interventions will affect the impact that the intervention may have. This partly explains why, when randomized trials have been undertaken, they usually find no significant effect, whereas non-randomized studies often find significant benefits. It is probably because those who choose to participate recognize and accept the need to improve, which, in itself, may be more important than the actual intervention. Thus it cannot be known whether or not any observed effect in non-randomized studies can be attributed to the intervention being evaluated (was it the intervention or the participants' attitudes and beliefs?).

Even more challenging than establishing the effectiveness of quality improvement interventions is determining their efficiency (cost-benefit). The latter will be dependent on assumptions that must be made about the sustainability of any improvements. If the improvements in quality are permanent, the benefits continue to accrue for many years and will be huge, whereas the cost is limited to the initial intervention. The cost-benefit will depend almost entirely on the sustainability of any effect rather than the size of the effect.

Regardless of the approaches described in this chapter, a few general insights about quality improvement can be made. It is more likely to be successful if:

- The cause of poor quality is correctly diagnosed (e.g. lack of knowledge, perverse incentives, over-complicated clinical pathway for patients).
- It has the support and involvement of the most respected opinion leaders in the clinical area.

- Participants recognize the need for change.
- There is a sense of ownership by those whose behaviour needs to change.
- The focus is on improving quality rather than reducing costs (even if the latter is also a benefit).
- A combination of approaches is used.
- The methods used are changed every so often to ensure persistence of the change.

Although accounts of quality improvement interventions (including most of the content of this chapter) tend to focus on the technical approaches available (such as scientific evidence/guidelines, quality assessment data, monitoring mechanisms), of equal importance to successful improvement are the relational aspects (Dixon-Woods et al., 2012; Health Foundation, 2009). These include such aspects as: the culture of the organization, which needs to support and encourage staff to be self-critical and enquiring rather than blaming and punishing poor quality; leadership at every level from clinical teams and wards to the board of the organization – 'ward-to-board' involvement; staff engagement and motivation to want to improve and provide a better service; transparency about the quality achieved, shared not only with staff but also with patients and the public; good communication within the organization and with patients; and focusing on the needs and experiences of patients, so-called patient-centred care. Recognition and attention to these aspects will ensure the quality of care will improve even if it is not possible to identify and measure the contributions of each specific intervention.

Summary

You may be wondering, in what way does quality improvement differ from the key management task of bringing about transformational change of health services? The answer is that it doesn't. Alongside financial management, quality improvement is one of the two key tasks of management.

You have seen how there is a wide variety of quality improvement approaches available and that these can be considered within five categories. You have learnt about the potential uses and benefits of different approaches, and how, whichever approach is adopted, its success will depend on the culture, values, and leadership of the health care organization.

References

Batalden, P.B. and Davidoff, F. (2007) What is 'quality improvement' and how can it transform healthcare?, *Quality and Safety in Health Care*, 16 (1): 2–3.

Biller-Andorno, N. and Lee, T.H. (2013) Ethical physician incentives – from carrots and sticks to shared purpose, *New England Journal of Medicine*, 368 (11): 980–2.

Black, N. (2015) To do the service no harm: the dangers of quality assessment, *Journal of Health Services Research and Policy*, 20 (2): 65–6.

Cayton, H. and Webb, K. (2014) The benefits of a 'right-touch' approach to health care regulation, *Journal of Health Services Research and Policy*, 19 (4): 198–9.

Dixon-Woods, M., McNicol, S. and Martin, G. (2012) Ten challenges in improving quality in healthcare: lessons from the Health Foundation's programme evaluations and relevant literature, *BMJ Quality and Safety*, 21 (10): 876–84.

Elwyn, G., Laitner, S., Coulter, A., Walker, E., Watson, P. and Thomson, R. (2010) Implementing shared decision-making in the NHS, *British Medical Journal*, 341: c5146.

Gopalan, S.S., Mutasa, R., Friedman, J. and Das, A. (2014) Health sector demand-side financial incentives in low- and middle-income countries: a systematic review on demand- and supply-side effects, *Social Science and Medicine*, 100: 72–83.

Health Foundation (2009) *What Works to Improve Quality in Healthcare?* London: Health Foundation.

Hoffman, A. and Emanuel, E.J. (2013) Reengineering US health care, *Journal of the American Medical Association*, 309 (7): 661–2.

O'Connor, A.M., Bennett, C.L., Stacey, D., Barry, M., Col, N.F., Eden, K.B. et al. (2009) Decision aids for people facing health treatment or screening decisions. *Cochrane Database of Systematic Reviews*, 3: CD001431.

Glossary

Accreditation: Voluntary schemes run by independent bodies assessing attributes of an organization largely based on structural characteristics rather than processes or outcomes.

Adverse selection: When a party enters into an agreement in which they can use their own private information to the disadvantage of another party.

Agency theory (or principal-agent theory): Describes the problems that arise under conditions of asymmetric information between two parties, the principal and the agent.

Ambulatory care: Health care provided to patients without admitting them to hospital such as general practice, out-patient clinics, and day care.

Bureaucracy: A formal type of organization involving hierarchy, impersonality, continuity, and expertise.

Capitation payment: A predetermined amount of money per member of a defined population served by the third party payer, given to a provider to deliver specific services.

Case-mix: The mix of cases (patients) that a provider cares for that will inevitably influence the outcome of care (e.g. age, severity, co-morbidity).

Case series: Study of a series of cases to identify common or recurring features.

Case study: Observation and analysis of a single case to generate a hypothesis.

Catastrophic expenditure: Expenditure at such a high level as to force households to reduce spending on other basic goods (e.g. food or water), to sell assets or to incur high levels of debt, and ultimately to risk impoverishment.

Clinical guidelines: Advice based on the best available research evidence and the consensus view of clinicians.

Clinical or professional judgement: The decision taken by a clinician as to whether or not a patient has a normative need.

Clinical pathway: The route or journey a patient follows from lay referral to treatment.

Community participation: A process by which individuals or groups assume responsibility for health matters of their community.

Community-rated contribution: Insurance premiums that are based on pooled risk of the entire community rather than the claims experience or personal level of risk of an individual.

Compliance: The extent to which a patient follows professional advice.

Confounder: Characteristics of patients that are associated both with their likelihood of being treated and the likelihood of the outcome (e.g. age, severity).

Consensus development: A set of explicit formal methods for developing and establishing the collective views of a group when faced with uncertainty.

Consumerism: A social movement promoting and representing user interests in health services.

Co-production: The combination of professionals and patients in their clinical management, particularly for long-term conditions.

Corporate rationalizers: A contemporary approach to management in which the organization (corporation) attempts to dominate professional autonomy through the use of measurement and data.

Cream-skimming (or cherry-picking): When an insurance scheme enrols a disproportionate number of individuals who present a lower than average risk of ill health or high-cost care.

Critical incident inquiry: A set of procedures used for collecting direct observations of actions that have critical significance and meet methodically defined criteria.

Culture: The values, beliefs, and attitudes associated with a social system.

Demand: Expressed need for health services.

Disability (functional status): The impact of an impairment on the patient's ability to function.

Discourse: The way language is used in a particular area.

Disease: A condition, which, judged by the prevailing culture, is painful or disabling and deviates from either the statistical norm or from some idealized status.

Diseases: Patterns of factors (symptoms, signs) that occur in many people in more or less the same way.

DRG (Diagnosis Related Group)/HRG (Healthcare Resource Group): A case-mix classification scheme that provides a means of relating the number and type of acute in-patients treated in a hospital to the resources required by the hospital.

Empathy: A response that demonstrates understanding and acceptance of the patient's feelings and concerns.

Encounter: The interaction of two or more people in a face-to-face meeting.

Environmental turbulence: The ever-changing external pressures on an organization and its managers such as legislation, the national economy, professional associations and trades unions, and public opinion.

Evidence-based medicine: The conscientious, explicit, and judicious use of current best evidence in making decisions about the care of individual patients.

Fee-for-service: Payment mechanism whereby providers receive a specific amount of money for each service provided.

Felt need: A person's subjective assessment of their need (self-assessment).

Formal care: Care provided by trained, paid professionals usually in a formal setting.

Global workforce crisis: A shortage of health workers across the world that has been exacerbated by the global demand for health care.

Health-related quality of life (handicap, well-being): The impact of disability (functional status) on a person's social functioning, partly determined by their environment and circumstances (e.g. housing, economic status).

Health services research (HSR): A multidisciplinary activity to improve the quality, organization, and management of health services. HSR is not itself a discipline.

Holism: The conceptualization of a system as a whole and the belief that the whole is greater than the sum of its parts.

Hospital-wide standardized mortality ratio: The number of deaths in a hospital compared with the number that would be expected (based on the average performance of all hospitals).

Hybrid professionals: A professional embodying the working practices and principles of two different roles in their work.

Iatrogenesis: Disease or harm resulting from health care interventions.

Ideal type: A hypothetical model of a complex real phenomenon that emphasizes its most salient features.

Ideology: A set of beliefs, values, and attitudes used to justify and legitimize power.

Impairment: The physical signs of the condition (pathology), usually measured objectively by clinicians.

Inputs: The resources needed by a system.

Inverse care law: The observation that availability of care appears to be inversely related to need.

Lay care: Care provided by lay people who have received no formal training and are not paid. It includes self-care and care provided by relatives, friends, and self-help groups.

Litigation: Legal action taken by patients against health care providers for alleged malpractice.

Medical cosmology: The study of medical paradigms.

Medicalization: The preference for defining problems as 'medical' and thus subject to the involvement of medical practitioners (also referred to as medical imperialism).

Medical paradigm: The prevailing thoughts and knowledge about health and disease.

Moral hazard: When one of the parties to an agreement has an incentive, after the agreement is made, to act in a manner that brings additional benefits to themselves at the expense of the other party.

Normative need: A professional assessment of a person's need based on objective measures (professional or biomedical assessment).

Outcomes: Change in status as a result of the system processes (in the health services context, the change in health status as a result of care).

Outputs: A combination of the processes and outcomes that constitute the total production of a system.

Pathological: Form or function that is deemed to be abnormal.

Patient experience: The patient's views of the humanity of the care they receive, covering such aspects as respect and dignity, receiving information, waiting times, etc. Seeks to be objective, avoiding patient's subjective expectations.

Patient reported outcome measures (PROMs): Outcomes reported by patients using questionnaires that may be generic (general aspects of a person's health, such as mobility, sleeping, and appetite) or disease-specific (focused on a particular disease). Also referred to as patient reported outcomes (PROs).

Patient satisfaction: Patients' satisfaction with the humanity of care received. Influenced by a patient's expectations.

Payers: The people who provide funds to pay for health care.

Physiological: Referring to a bodily function (such as breathing) that is deemed to be 'normal'.

Pooling: The process of accumulating and managing revenue to ensure that the contributors to the pool share risks.

Power: The ability to influence – and in particular to control – others, events, and resources.

Precision medicine: The application of specific knowledge of individual variability in the choice of prevention and treatment strategies.

Primary care: Formal care that is the first point of contact for people. It is usually general rather than specialized and provided in the community.

Processes: The use of resources or the activity within a system.

Profession: An occupation based on specified knowledge and training and regulated standards of performance.

Professional autonomy: The freedom that professionals have to make decisions without being 'accountable' to their employers or the state.

Professionalization: A process whereby an occupation achieves the more independent status of a profession.

Progressive: A financing mechanism whereby groups with a higher income contribute a higher percentage of their income than do groups with a lower income.

Prospective payment: Paying providers before any care is delivered, usually on the basis of capitation payments or contracts.

Providers: Organizations (hospitals, health centres) or individuals (community nurses) who provide formal or informal care.

Public trust: The expectation that professionals will be knowledgeable and competent and will behave in the patient's best interest with beneficence, fairness, and integrity.

Purchasers: Those who purchase health services from providers on behalf of those eligible to use health care.

Purchasing: The process of allocating funds to health care providers.

Quality care: Care that is safe, effective, humane, equitable, and sustainable.

Quality management: A systematic approach to quality of care that encompasses defining, assessing, and improving the quality of health services.

Random variation: Statistical differences that occur by chance and are inevitable when counting events.

Redesign (re-engineer): Changes to the way services are organized at a micro-level (e.g. a health centre, ward, clinic).

Reductionism: Consideration of the component parts rather than the whole organism or organization.

Regressive: A financing mechanism whereby groups with a lower income contribute a higher percentage of their income than do groups with a higher income.

Relative need: Comparison between needs of individuals with similar conditions or between needs of populations living in similar areas.

Reliability: The extent to which an instrument (e.g. clinical test, questionnaire) produces consistent results.

Reprofessionalization: A change in the nature of how the (medical) profession is viewed.

Responsiveness: The extent to which an instrument (e.g. clinical test, questionnaire) detects real changes in the state of health of a person.

Retrospective case record review: Patients' medical records are reviewed to determine if there were any acts of commission (e.g. giving the wrong drug) or of omission (e.g. failing to carry out a test) that caused harm.

Retrospective payment: Paying providers for any work they have undertaken, with no agreement in advance.

Revenue collection: The process by which the health system raises funds from households, organizations, and external sources such as donors.

Risk (case-mix) adjustment: A statistical process to make allowance for any difference in case-mix between providers when comparing their performance.

Risk-rated contribution: Insurance premium adjusted to the level of the individual's or group's risk of illness, expected future cost of health care use or past claims experience.

Secondary care: Specialized care that often can only be accessed by being referred by a primary care worker. It is usually provided in local hospitals.

Self-help groups: Groups of unpaid, self-taught people that offer solutions to health problems in a lay setting, based on mutual support between persons experiencing similar conditions.

Shared decision-making: The sharing of decisions between professionals and patients, which can be aided by computer software incorporating probabilities of different outcomes and patients' utilities.

Social role: A set of ideas and actions that let individuals behave according to expected social norms.

Standardized mortality ratio: An indicator of the frequency of deaths in a population that takes into account the age and sex structure of the population.

Surveillance medicine: The widespread monitoring of the population for symptoms of disease or for established conditions.

Sustainability: The capacity of health services/systems to endure financially, socially, and environmentally.

System: A model of a whole entity, reflecting the relationship between its elements at different levels of complexity.

Systematic review: A review of the literature that uses an explicit approach to searching, selecting, and combining the relevant studies.

Systematic variation: Statistical differences that cannot be accounted for by the inevitable random variations that occur when counting events.

Tertiary care: Highly specialized care that often can only be accessed by referral from secondary care. It is usually provided in national or regional hospitals.

Total quality management: An approach to quality improvement that involves the commitment of all members of an organization to meeting the needs of its external and internal customers.

Universal health coverage: When all people can use the promotive, preventive, curative, rehabilitative, and palliative health services they need, of sufficient quality to be effective, while also ensuring that the use of these services does not expose the user to financial hardship.

Use: Utilization of health services that are actually provided.

Utilization rate: A measure of health service use.

Validity: The extent to which an instrument (e.g. clinical test, questionnaire) measures what it intends to measure.

Index

abnormal, changes in recognition of 43, 44
accountability 5, 197–8
   current focus on 10–12, 209
accreditation 226, 235, 240
adverse selection 81, 92, 240
Agency for Health Research and Quality (ARHQ)
      202
agency relationships 159–60
agency theory 158, 240
allocation mechanisms 95
alternative medicine 25, 68–9
   see also traditional medicine/healers
ambulatory care 61, 240
   hospitalization for ambulatory care–sensitive
         conditions 119, 120
American Medical Association 65
anthroposophic medicine 57
Armstrong, D. 56
Arnstein, S.R. 145, 146
Asher, R. 59
aspects of health status 183–5
assessment
   current focus on 10–12, 209
   needs assessment 112–18
   self-assessment 38
autonomy see professional autonomy

bedside medicine 55
Beijing Declaration 68
Bernhart, M. 136–9
biomedical (professional) assessment
      38, 39
biomedical model 16
   dangers of the biomedical paradigm 58–9
Black, N. 7, 14–19, 125, 188–90
Bond, A. 180
Bonnerjea, L. 26
boundary disputes 73
Bowling, A. 151–2
British Lying-In Hospital 209
Brook, R.H. 214–15
bureaucracy 133, 140, 142–3, 240

   professional 67–8
Busse, R. 166–9

Calnan, M. 135
capitation payments 158, 162–3, 240
care options 26–31
   see also formal care; lay care
care-seeking behaviour 26–31
case-based payments 165–9
case-mix 208, 212–16, 240
case studies 52, 59, 240
Cashin, C. 170
catastrophic expenditure 81, 89, 240
categories of care 128–30
categorization of diseases 43–5, 53
   importance of classification 45–6
Centre for Reviews and Dissemination 204–5
certification 234, 235
charters 146
checklist-based observation 220–1
cherry-picking (cream-skimming) 81, 92,
      167–8, 241
choice 144–5
citizens 134, 147–55
Cleary, P. 191–4
clinical databases 219
clinical guidelines 196, 199, 202–7, 229, 240
clinical iceberg 110, 111
clinical (professional) judgement 17, 107, 240
   cultural differences 48–9
   need, demand and use 108, 112, 126–8
clinical-management roles 68, 75
clinical pathway 226, 232–3, 240
clinical research 52, 59, 240
Cochrane Collaboration 204
code of ethics/practice 63
Codman, E.A. 209
collaborative, localized, enabling approach
      181, 182
collaboratives 234
collecting organizations 94
collective decision-making 147–55

communication with patients 135
community empowerment 145, 146
community health insurance 93–4, 98, 101
community leaders' preferences 154–5
community model of health care delivery 134, 147–55
community participation 133, 134, 147–55, 240
community-rated contributions 81, 91, 92, 93, 240
complementary medicine 25, 68–9
  see also traditional medicine/healers
completeness of data 212
compliance 134, 140, 144, 240
confounders 208, 213, 240
consensus development 196, 206–7, 241
consistency of definitions 211–12
consumerism 72, 134–7, 144, 241
consumers 134, 144–7
continuity 142
contribution mechanisms 85–94
  community health insurance 93–4, 98, 101
  mandatory health insurance 85, 89–91, 97
  medical savings accounts 94
  out-of-pocket payments 85–9, 98
  private health insurance 90, 91–3, 98
  taxation 85, 89, 90, 96–7, 100–1
co-payments 85–9, 232
co-production 226, 229, 241
corporate elite 75
corporate rationalizers 3, 13, 18, 241
corporate sector 46
cost 5–6, 179
  era of cost containment 10–11, 12, 13
cost-benefit 237
cost sharing (user charges) 85–6, 88–9, 93
Cots, F. 168
Coulter, A. 143, 147
Crawford, M.J. 152–3
cream-skimming (cherry-picking) 81, 92, 167–8, 241
critical incident inquiries 208, 210, 241
cultural norms 140, 141–2
culture 37, 41–2, 241
  and disease 47–50

data quality 123, 211–12
Davies, H. 197–8
decision-making
  public input 147–55
  shared 227, 229–31, 244

defensive practice 236–7
defining good quality services 196–207
  evidence-based medicine 196, 199–201, 241
  evidence-based policy-making 201–2
  guidelines 196, 199, 202–7, 229, 240
  trust and accountability 197–8
demand 107–32, 241
  demand-side factors and variations in use 123–6
  need, supply and 113–18
diagnosis related groups (DRGs) 158, 166–9, 241
Dickens, C. 8
direct payments 85, 88, 98
direct taxes 89, 90, 96–7
disability (functional status) 177, 184–5, 186, 191, 193, 241
discourse 52, 54, 241
  rationale for studying changes in 54–7
disease(s) 37–51, 241
  categorization 43–5, 53
  culture and 47–50
  defining 38–43
  importance of classification 45–6
  name changes 43
  severity and service use 125
disease mongering 46
disease-specific measures 186–7
Dixon, A. 124
Dixon, J. 153–4
Donabedian, A. 182
dumping 167–8

E-scaped medicine 57
Economist, The 217–18
education 229–31
effective care 128, 129–30
effectiveness 73, 179, 211
  challenges when assessing 211–16
efficiency 237
elections 6
eligibility for treatment 45
elites, professional 75–6
Ellwood, P. 11–12
Elston, M.A. 26
Elwyn, G. 230
emotional support 24
empathy 134, 135, 241
employment 90
employment rights 45

encounters 134, 241
  staff-patient encounters 135–44
engagement in quality assessment 222–4
Engelhardt, H.T. 58
Ensor, T. 160, 161
environment
  environmental turbulence 3, 14, 15–16,
    18–19, 201–2, 241
  internal 15
  physical 8
environmental limits 181–2
equity 179, 211
  in health care financing 96–8
Europe 166–9
EuroQuol (EQ-5D) 187
evidence-based medicine (EBM) 196, 199–201,
    241
evidence-based policy–making 201–2
exit interviews 221
expansion, era of 10, 12
expectations 197–8
expenditure on health care 5–6, 89, 90
experience
  combining research evidence with 205–7
  measures of patients' experiences 188–94,
    210–11
  patient experience 178, 243
Expert Patients Programme 144
expertise 63, 72, 142
  individual clinical expertise 199–201
  technical 65
external clinical evidence 199–201
external pressures 15–16, 18–19

fee-for-service payments 158, 161, 162, 164–5,
    241
felt need 38, 39, 108–9, 110, 111, 118, 241
Ferket, B.S. 205–6
finance see funding
financial incentives 231–2
  payment mechanisms and 161, 162, 163,
    164, 165, 166, 169–72
Finland 146
fiscal space 89
Florin, D. 153–4
formal care 5, 14, 21–33, 241
  demand for 111
  lay care vs 23–5
  workers' attitudes towards lay care 31–2
Foucault, M. 54

France 48, 49
Franco, L. 220–1
Freidson, E. 64, 70, 71
Fry, J. 29
functional status (disability) 177, 184–5, 186,
    191, 193, 241
functionalism 69–70, 71, 141–2
funding 8, 14, 81–103
  collecting organizations 94
  contribution mechanisms 85–94
  equity in 96–8
  functions and goals of 82–3
  pooling of funds 82, 95–6, 100, 101
  progressive 82, 96–8, 243
  public participation in decision-making 148,
    149–50, 151–2
  regressive 82, 96, 97, 98, 244
  revenue collection 82, 84–94, 244
  sources of 84–5
  universal health coverage 82, 83–4, 95,
    98–101, 245

Gabbay, J. 113–17
gender 66–7
  see also women
General Medical Council 64–5
generic measures 186–7
genetics 56
global budgets 169
global workforce crisis 61, 76–8, 241
Glover, J.A. 126
governance elite 75
government 15–16, 18
  funding of health services 14, 85, 86, 89,
    100–1
  taxation 85, 89, 90, 96–7, 100–1
government health centres and hospitals 27–8,
    30
GP referral rates 119, 127
Green, J. 74
Groves, E.W. 209
guidelines 196, 199, 202–7, 229, 240
Guidelines International Network 202

Hannan, E. 213–15
Harding, S. 135
Hart, J.T. 126
Hawker, G.A. 125–6
heads of households 154–5
health care professionals 5, 8, 13, 16, 61–80

clinical judgement *see* clinical (professional) judgement
comparing medicine and nursing 66–7
defining a professional 62–4
engaging in quality assessment 222–4
global workforce crisis 61, 76–8, 241
hybrid professionals 62, 74–6, 242
international context 68–9
medical profession *see* medical profession
reprofessionalization 62, 74–6, 244
role of managers 67–8
skill mix 76
staff-patient interactions 135–44
health expenditure 5–6, 89, 90
health insurance 85, 89–94
community 93–4, 98, 101
mandatory 85, 89–91, 97
private 90, 91–3, 98
health-related quality of life 177, 184–5, 186, 242
health services research (HSR) 4, 14–19, 242
healthcare resource groups (HRGs) 158, 166–9
hierarchy 142
historical background
of the health service 7–9
to quality assessment 209–10
holism 52, 55, 56, 57, 242
hospital-wide standardized mortality ratios (SMRs) 209, 218–20, 242
hospitalization for ambulatory care-sensitive conditions 119, 120
hospital(s)
architecture 16
categories of care 129–30
clinicians 58–9
medicine 55
payments to 163–9
humours of the body 55
hybrid professionals 62, 74–6, 242
hypothecated taxation 89

iatrogenesis 38, 70, 242
ideal type 62, 63, 242
ideals 41, 42
ideology 62, 63, 242
opposition to medical profession 73
Illich, I. 70, 71
illness behaviour 123, 125–6

impairment 177, 184–5, 186, 242
incentives
financial *see* financial incentives
perverse 213–14, 215
quality improvement 231–2
inclusion/exclusion criteria 204–5
independent nurse practitioners 66
index measure of health system quality 216–17
indirect taxes 89, 97
individual clinical expertise 199–201
individual practitioner payments 161–3
informal payments 86
information asymmetry 159–60
information provision 24, 135
information sources 115–16
inputs 4, 6–7, 182, 183, 242
see also diseases; funding; health care professionals; medical paradigms
inspection 235
institutions
engaging in quality assessment 222–4
payments to 163–9
rigidity 227
see also hospitals
insurance
compensation 45
health *see* health insurance
intermediate outcome 187
international migration 76–8
inter-observer (inter-rater) reliability 187–8
intra-observer reliability 188
inverse care law 107, 126–8, 242

Jegers, M. 164
Jenkinson, C. 188–90
Jewson, N. 55
Jones, L. 74

Kakwani index 97
King, L. 39–42
knowledge base 63, 72
knowledge elite 75
Kutzin, J. 83, 99, 100–1

laboratory medicine 56
ladder of participation 145, 146
Langenbrunner, J. 160, 161, 165
language 53–4
Last, J. 110–11

law profession 63
lay care 5, 14, 21–33, 242
  changing nature of 31
  demand for 111
  extent of 25–31
  vs formal care 23–5
  formal care workers' attitudes towards 31–2
lay knowledge movement 73
lay referral mechanisms 29
Le Grand, J. 124
Lean production 234
legal action 226, 236–7, 242
legislation on patients' rights 146
levels of analysis 216–20
levels of health care 22–3
Levin, L.S. 28–9
Levinson, W. 135
licensing 234
limitation 64
line-item budgets 163–4
litigation 226, 236–7, 242
local interests 15–16, 18
local taxation 89
Lomas, J. 147–51
low-income countries
  quality assessment 220–1
  universal health coverage 98–101
Lupton, D. 74, 147

Mackenbach, J.P. 123, 124
macro level 216–18
managerial elite 75
managerialism 72, 74, 75
managers 67–8
  clinical-management roles 68, 75
  managerial-professional hybrid 74–6
mandatory health insurance 85, 89–91, 97
markets 14, 64
  market-driven model of health care delivery
    134, 144–7
Marxism 70
Medicaid 10, 12
medical cosmology 53, 242
medical expansion 70, 71
medical-industrial complex 16, 19
medical knowledge 37–51
  aspects of 53
  categorization of diseases 43–5
  importance of disease classification 45–6
medical paradigms 52–60, 242

dangers of the biomedical/clinical paradigm
    58–9
  importance of language 53–4
  reasons for studying shifts in 54–7
medical pluralism 73
medical profession 63–79
  agency relationships 159–60
  compared with the nursing profession 66–7
  and managers 68
  power of 64–5
  reprofessionalization 74–6
  role in society 69–71
  threats to 71–3
  see also health care professionals
medical savings accounts 94
medicalization 38, 46–7, 70, 242
Medicare 10, 12, 171
meso level 218–20
met need 108, 109
middle-income countries
  quality assessment 220–1
  universal health coverage 98–101
migration, international 76–8
Mills, A. 97
Mintzberg, H. 67
Mol, A. 142
monopoly 63, 64–5, 70
  threats to 72
moral hazard 82, 90, 91–3, 242
morbidity rates 116
mortality 183, 184, 186, 192
Mountford, J. 222–4
Moynihan, R. 46
Msiska, R. 26–31

National Clinical Guideline Centre 202
National Institute for Health and Clinical
    Excellence (NICE) 202
National Institutes of Health 10
need 107–32
  demand, supply and 113–18
  felt 38, 39, 108–9, 110, 111, 118, 241
  met 108, 109
  normative 38, 39, 108–9, 110, 118, 242
  relative 107, 110, 244
  unfelt 109, 110, 111, 112
  unmet 108, 109
  and variations in use 123–6
needs assessment 112–18
negotiated order 67

Nettleton, S. 135
Neuberger, J. 125
new diseases 43
Nightingale, F. 209
nineteenth-century hospital medicine 55
Nissel, M. 26
nominal group technique 206–7
Noordegraaf, M. 74
normal functions 43
normative need 38, 39, 108–9, 110, 118, 242
norms
    cultural 140, 141–2
    statistical 39–40, 41
nursing profession 66–7

Obama, B. 57
objective explanations of disease 38–43
objective measures of health 190–4
observation 41, 220–1
O'Connor, A.M. 230–1
O'Donnell, C.A. 127
O'Donnell, O. 97
OECD countries 170
Omoigui, N.A. 214
Onwujekwe, O. 154–5
Oregon process 148
organizing professionalism 74
out-of-pocket payments 85–9, 98
outcomes 4, 6–7, 11, 182–94, 242
    approaches to measurement 186
    aspects of health to measure 183–5
    patient-reported outcome measures 178,
        186–94, 243
    risk-adjusted outcome rates 213–16
    see also defining good quality services; quality
        assessment; quality of health services;
        quality improvement
outcomes management 11–12
outputs 4, 242
over-reporting of risk factors 214, 215
overtreatment 167–8

pain 41
Palència, L. 124
Parsons, T. 69–70, 141
pathological form/function 38, 242
patient-centred care 143–4
patient-day payment mechanism 165
patient-doctor agency relationship 159–60
patient experience 178, 243

patient reported experience measures (PREMs)
    188–94, 210–11
patient reported outcome measures (PROMs)
    178, 186–94, 243
patient satisfaction 178, 189, 243
    in developing countries 136–9
patients 13
    changes in the role of 143–4, 147
    users as 134, 135–44
pay for performance (P4P) 169–72
Payer, L. 48–9
payers 4, 10–11, 16, 243
payments see provider payments
Pencheon, D. 180–2
per-diem payment system 165
perceived health 191–2
performance-based payments 169–72
perverse incentives 213–14, 215
Peters, M. 25–6
physical environment 8
physiological function 38, 243
plan, do, study, act cycle 233
policy-making
    evidence-based 201–2
    public participation 147–55
political elite 75
pooling 92, 95–6, 100, 101, 243
population-based payment 160–1
population-based utilization rates 118, 119–20
power 62, 64, 243
    community empowerment 145, 146
    incentives to strengthen consumer power
        145–7
    language and 54
    of the medical profession 64–5
    relative 140
practical assistance 24
practice elite 75
precision medicine 53, 56–7, 243
Precision Medicine Catapult 57
preference-sensitive care 128–30
pre-nineteenth-century medicine 55
previously rare conditions, uncovering of 43,
    44–5
primary care 21, 22, 23, 243
    categories of care 129–30
principal-agent theory 158, 159–60
priority-setting 148–55
private health insurance 90, 91–3, 98
privileges 141

processes 4, 6–7, 182–3, 211, 214–15, 243
  see also demand; need; provider payments;
    use; users of health care
professional assessment 38, 39
professional autonomy 4, 18, 243
  medical profession 69–71, 72
professional bureaucracy 67–8
professional elites 75–6
professional judgement see clinical (professional)
    judgement
professional-managerial hybrid 74–6
professional model of health care delivery 134,
    135–44
professional organizations 18, 73
professionalism 74, 75
professionalization 62, 63, 70, 77, 243
professions 62, 243
  defining a professional 62–4
  health care see health care professionals
progressive financing 82, 96–8, 243
proportional financing 96
prospective payment 4, 10, 243
provider interviews 221
provider payments 158–73
  individual practitioners 161–3
  institutions 163–9
  performance-based 169–72
  prospective payments 4, 10, 243
  retrospective payments 4, 244
  typology of payment mechanisms 160–1
providers 4, 243
psychosomatic medicine 57
public, the 16
public health facilities 27–8, 30
public participation 145, 146
  users as communities and citizens 147–55
public trust 197–8, 243
'pull' factors 77, 78
purchasers 4, 243
purchasing 82–3, 243
'push' factors 77, 78

qualitative quality assessment 210–11
quality assessment 208–25
  challenges when assessing effectiveness
    211–16
  engaging clinicians and institutions 222–4
  history 209–10
  levels of analysis 216–20
  in low- and middle-income countries 220–1

range of methods needed 210–11
quality care 178, 243
quality of health services 162, 163, 177–95
  approaches to measurement 186
  aspects of health to measure 183–5
  defining quality 178–82
  measuring patients' experiences and outcomes
    188–90
  selection of a measure 186–8
  structure, processes and outcomes 182–3
  subjective and objective measures 190–4
quality improvement 226–39
  education 229–31
  effectiveness of 237–8
  incentives 231–2
  legal action 226, 236–7, 242
  mapping interventions 227–8
  redesign 226, 232–4, 244
  regulation 234–6
quality of life, health-related 177, 184–5, 186,
    242
quality management 178, 244
  cycle 194–5
quantitative quality assessment 210–11

random variation 107, 123, 244
randomized controlled trials 237
rationing 109, 150–1
readmissions
  frequent 167–8
  rates 183
recognition of abnormal, changes in 43, 44
record reviews 209, 210, 221, 244
redesign (re-engineering) 226, 232–4, 244
reductionism 53, 56, 244
referral rates 119, 127
reform 9–13
regressive financing 82, 96, 97, 98, 244
regulation 234–6
regulatory capture 236
relationship with other professionals 64, 65
relative need 107, 110, 244
relative power 140
reliability 178, 187–8, 193, 194, 212, 244
religion 8
Relman, A. 9–13, 209
reluctance to challenge established views 59
repetitive strain injury 45
reprofessionalization 62, 74–6, 244
research

clinical 52, 59, 240
creating guidelines 204–7
evidence-based medicine 196, 199–201, 241
evidence-based policy-making 201–2
health services research 4, 14–19, 242
resource allocation 95
responsiveness 178, 189, 244
retirement rates 43
retrospective case record reviews 209, 210, 221, 244
retrospective payment 4, 244
revalidation 234
revenue collection 82, 84–94, 244
review question 204–5
rewards 24
risk (case-mix) adjustment 209, 212–16, 244
risk-rated contributions 82, 91, 92–3, 244
risk selection 91–3
Robinson, J. 66
Roemer, M. 128
routine work 140
Rwanda 101
  P4P 170, 171–2

Sackett, D.L. 199–201
safety 210
salary payments 161–2
Savedoff, W. 99–100
Schaeffer, A. 26
screening 109, 112
secondary care 21, 22, 23, 244
self-assessment 38
self-care 28–9
self-help groups 22, 32, 244
self-help movements 73
self-interest 70, 71
self-management programmes 229
service availability 126, 128
service-based payment 160–1, 162
service-based utilization rates 118, 119
service recipients 149, 150–1
services to offer decisions 149, 150, 151–2
setting 24, 58
Shahian, D. 218
shared decision-making 227, 229–31, 244
Shaw, G.B. 70
Shojana, K. 222–4
Short Form 36 (SF36) 187
sick leave 141, 142
sick role 141, 142

Sinyor, J.K. 136
Six sigma 234
skills mix 76
Smith, K. 26
Smith, R. 45–6
social attitudes 8
social care 26
social construct, disease as 43
social cost 29–30
social roles 134, 141–2, 244
social security payments 232
social security rights 46
socio-behavioural incentives 231
socio-demographic changes 8
socio-economic status 123–4
staff organizations 16, 18
staff-patient interactions 135–44
  compliance and 140
  factors influencing 136–9
  societal forces shaping 140–3
standardization of skills 67–8
standardized mortality ratios (SMRs) 125, 245
  hospital-wide 209, 218–20, 242
statistical norms 39–40, 41
statistical process control 234
statistics 123
status 64, 66–7, 71
Stevens, A. 113–17
stigmatization 30
stoics 38
Strauss, A. 67
Strong, P. 66
structure 182–3
sub-division of disease categories 43, 44
subjective explanations of disease 38–43
subjective measures of health 190–4
subjugation 64
supplier-induced demand 112
supply
  need, demand and 113–18
  supply-side factors and variations in use 126–8
supply-sensitive care 128, 129–30
surgery 16–18, 230–1
  rates of 48, 127
surveillance medicine 53, 56, 245
sustainability 178, 179–82, 245
Sustainable Development Goals 83
symptoms 184–5, 186, 193
systematic reviews 197, 204–5, 245

systematic variation 108, 123, 245
systems approach 3–20, 245
  contemporary challenges 13–14
  factors influencing change and reform 9–13
  health services research and services
      management 14–19
  historical factors role in shaping health
      services 7–9

targets 235–6
taxation 85, 89, 90, 96–7, 100–1
technical expertise 65
technology 8, 57
  harnessing and sustainability 181, 182
tertiary care 22, 23, 245
time-based payment 160–1
total quality management 227, 228, 245
traditional medicine/healers 25, 27, 30, 57,
      68–9
training 24, 63
trust 71
  public 197–8, 243
twentieth-century laboratory medicine 56
twenty-first-century precision medicine 56–7

uncertainty 65
unfelt need 109, 110, 111, 112
unintended consequences 167–9
United Kingdom (UK) 17, 50, 57, 77, 205–6
  General Medical Council 64–5
  historical factors shaping health services 7, 8
  hospitalization for ambulatory care–sensitive
      conditions 119, 120
  HRGs 166, 167, 168
  lack of lay care for older people 31
  Medical Act 1858 64
  National Clinical Guideline Centre 202
  NICE 202
  Quality and Outcomes Framework (QOF) 171
United States of America (USA) 17, 48, 57,
      76–7, 205–6
  Affordable Care Act (Obamacare) 6
  ARHQ 202
  DRGs 166, 167
  factors influencing change and reform in
      health care 10–12

Premier Ltd Hospital Quality Incentive
      Demonstration (PHQID) 171
  rates of common surgical procedures 127
universal health coverage 82, 95, 245
  movement 83–4
  progress towards 98–101
unmet need 108, 109
upcoding 167–8
use 108–9, 118–30, 245
  causes of variations in use 120–8
  conceptual model of need, demand and 108–9
  unwarranted variation and categories of care
      128–30
use/need ratio 124–5
user charges (cost sharing) 85–6, 88–9, 93
users of health care 13, 133–57
  as communities and citizens 134, 147–55
  as consumers 134, 144–7
  as patients 134, 135–44
utilization rates 108, 115, 118–20, 245

validity 178, 187, 193, 194, 205, 212, 245
value-based health care 232
Van Doorslaer, E. 123–4
variations in use see use

Wagstaff, A. 97
waiting lists 17–18, 115, 116
Waring, J. 75
wealth 64
Weber, M. 63, 142
Wennberg, J. 127, 128–9
Wiley, C. 165
Williams, S.J. 135
women
  lay carers 25, 26
  STD patients 29, 30
World Health Organization (WHO) 76
  Congress on Traditional Medicine 68
  functions of health financing 82–3
  Global Code of Practice on the International
      Recruitment of Health Personnel 77–8
  universal health coverage 83, 84
World Health Reports 76, 83, 90, 91, 216–17

Zander, A. 180